Atlas of Liver Transplantation

Chetana Lim • Chady Salloum • Daniel Azoulay

Atlas of Liver Transplantation

Springer

Chetana Lim
Chirurgie Hépato-Biliaire et
Transplantation hépatique
Hôpital Pitié-Salpêtrière
Paris, France

Daniel Azoulay
Centre Hépato-Biliaire
Hôpital Paul-Brousse
Villejuif, France

Chady Salloum
Centre Hépato-Biliaire
Hôpital Paul-Brousse
Villejuif, France

ISBN 978-3-031-85263-3 ISBN 978-3-031-85264-0 (eBook)
https://doi.org/10.1007/978-3-031-85264-0

This Springer imprint is published by the registered company Springer Nature Switzerland AG
The registered company address is: Gewerbestrasse 11, 6330 Cham, Switzerland

Foreword

After several hundred procedures in large animals, Thomas E. Starzl performed on March 1, 1963, a liver transplantation (LT) in three-year-old Eddy Solis, presenting end-stage secondary biliary cirrhosis due to extra-hepatic biliary atresia. Despite the extensive preparation of the Denver team, the procedure revealed itself to be tedious and . . . very dangerous: "the operative wound was exceedingly difficult to keep dry" . . . "the liver dissection was done with considerable difficulty."

After a moratorium of some years, LT activity was slowly picked up again. During the period March 1963 to April 1983, around 700 such procedures were done worldwide. The experiences from Denver-Pittsburgh, Hannover, Cambridge, and Groningen, accounting for 540 LTs, were the basis for the 1983 LT NIH Consensus conference. This meeting concluded that LT became "technically feasible" and "offered an alternative therapeutic approach which *may* prolong life in *some* patients suffering from severe liver disease that has progressed beyond reach of treatment." From then onwards, several hundreds of thousands of LTs have been performed successfully. The "impossible operation" became a daily reality thanks to the development of selective immunosuppression, the improvements of intra- and perioperative care, and, last but not least, the refinement of the surgical, procurement and transplantation, techniques.

It is many times forgotten that smooth post-transplant care starts with a perfect operation! Postoperative problems should be resolved intra-operatively! As the generation of surgeons who had the great opportunity to benefit from first-hand teaching, given by the liver transplant pioneers, is ending, it is important that past, good and bad (!), lessons and experiences from the operating theatre are not forgotten. Insufficient transmission of surgical knowledge is nowadays too many times the reason of a failing transplantation. This atlas helps to bridge this gap.

Besides the classical steps of organ procurement, total hepatectomy, and allograft implantation, this book very nicely documents particular aspects and situations, which are many times responsible for postoperative complications and even graft and recipient loss. The alternative hepatic artery and portal vein reconstructions (including anastomosis to renal artery and vein), the use of the umbilical vein (when installing veno-venous bypass or creating a temporary "portacaval" shunt), and the approach to different spontaneous portosystemic shunts are all good examples of this. The techniques of split LT, too many times forgotten as the "easiest" method to expand the allograft pool as well as the rarely used, auxiliary orthotopic LT, are also extensively highlighted. By giving attention to details, the once "unfinished LT product" becomes a finished one. Experiences from many centers worldwide have indeed shown that it becomes nowadays possible to perform LT without technical complications.

The 13 chapters of this book mirror the huge surgical knowledge, experience, and skills of the senior author, Professor Azoulay from the Centre Hépato-biliaire Henri Bismuth in Paris. Many next-generation liver transplant surgeons will without a doubt benefit from this very nicely illustrated book, bringing the operating room directly to their book shelves and vice versa. This *Atlas of Liver Transplantation* represents a great teaching tool that should be available in every liver transplantation center for both medical and paramedical staffs in order to allow them to better understand and perform the life-saving procedure that liver transplantation is.

Jan Lerut, MD, PhD
Past-director, Starzl Unit of Abdominal Transplantation
Past director, Université Catholique de Louvain (UCL)
Transplant Centre
Institute for Experimental and Clinical
Research (IREC), UCL
Brussels, Belgium

Foreword

Liver transplantation (LT) remains one of the most technically demanding surgical procedures, requiring a high level of medical and surgical expertise, especially in emergency settings. Initially described by Starzl in the 1960s, the procedure involved a standardized sequence of block clamping of the hepatic pedicle and inferior vena cava (IVC), enabling en bloc resection of the native liver, demanding rapid action to maintain hemodynamic tolerance, often necessitating veno-venous bypass.

While the classical LT procedure continues to be practiced globally, the 1980s saw a gradual transformation driven by the French school, who integrated their extensive hepatic surgery experience into LT. This led to the development of reduced and split-liver transplantation, extending the benefits of caval preservation and maintaining both caval and portal flow through temporary portocaval shunting. The possibility of transplant partial liver graft techniques revolutionized access to LT, particularly in countries with limited brain-dead donors, by enabling living donor transplantation. This evolution is masterfully showcased in a dedicated chapter on split-liver transplantation, illustrating the expertise of these three eminent French surgeons. Their insights, drawn from vast experience, resonate with the reality that no two LT procedures are identical, and meticulous planning is crucial to navigate challenges like parenchymal dysmorphisms, encapsulating peritonitis, and portal thromboses. This atlas stands as a testament to their profound expertise in classifying and overcoming these difficulties. It provides invaluable guidance on complex portal vein thrombosis reconstruction, alternative arterial revascularization using the recipient's splenic and renal arteries, and the management of large spontaneous portosystemic shunts.

This atlas is an admirable work of precision, capturing diverse surgical scenarios in striking photographs taken during urgent procedures. Like an astronaut viewing Earth, the absence of commentary facilitates direct, immediate observation of critical visual cues, resulting in both powerful pedagogical learning and the resonant recognition of surgical challenges.

Jacques Belghiti, MD

Former President of the International Liver Transplantation Society
Professor Emeritus at the University of Paris Cité and Former Head of the Liver Transplant Unit at Beaujon Clichy Hospital
Deputy Secretary of the Academy of Medicine
Paris, France

Preface

Liver transplantation still fascinates today because of its specificity, technical complexity, and challenges. Since Thomas Starzl performed the first liver transplant in 1963, few atlases have been published solely on liver transplantation. To address this, we first conceived this ambitious project in 2014 and began documenting and accumulating photographs in 2015. For three years, we captured this incredible surgical operation in both common and unusual ways, at times even using a smartphone.

The work is divided into 13 chapters that describe and illustrate the different stages of liver transplantation. Its primary objective is to portray common situations in liver transplantation: from graft harvesting to explantation of the native liver, portocaval anastomosis to biliary anastomosis.

The project, we believe, beautifully expresses the purpose of liver transplantation, demonstrating its splendors and helping to increase its understanding. Featuring more than 300 full-color photos, we omitted abbreviations or indications on the photos, intending to make the most beautiful and purely visual atlas available today.

The images in the Atlas, of course, do not cover all situations encountered in liver transplantation but, as Thomas Starzl said, liver transplantation is and will remain an "unfinished product."

Paris, France — Chetana Lim
Villejuif, France — Chady Salloum
Villejuif, France — Daniel Azoulay

Contents

1 Brain-Dead Donor Liver Procurement

During liver procurement, our approach is to perform a so-called *en-bloc technique* with significant bench dissection. This technique minimizes surgical injury rates and donor hepatectomy duration. The surgical technique is divided into warm and cold dissections. Warm dissection has the advantage of perfusion after confirming the vascular anatomy (Figs. 1.1, 1.2, 1.3, 1.4, 1.5, 1.6, 1.7, 1.8, 1.9, 1.10, 1.11, 1.12, 1.13, 1.14, 1.15, 1.16, 1.17, 1.18, 1.19, 1.20, 1.21, and 1.22). Cold dissection allows to reduce operative time and organ damage with rapid liver graft procurement (Figs. 1.23, 1.24, 1.25, 1.26, 1.27, 1.28, 1.29, 1.30, 1.31, 1.32, 1.33, 1.34, 1.35, 1.36, 1.37, 1.38, 1.39, 1.40, 1.41, 1.42, 1.43, 1.44, 1.45, 1.46, 1.47, 1.48, and 1.49).

After an abdominal midline incision with sternotomy, the distal aorta and inferior mesenteric vein are cannulated for hypothermic perfusion of the abdominal organs with ice-cold preservation solution. The organs are topically cooled with ice. The inferior vena cava is also cannulated to drain the effluent perfusate. Variable amounts of the liver and its vessels are dissected, and different amounts of perihepatic tissues procured with the liver are performed either during the warm phase or the cold phase, according to the surgeon's preferences and the donor's hemodynamic stability. Hilar dissection of the hepatic artery and cholecystectomy are not performed in this technique [1].

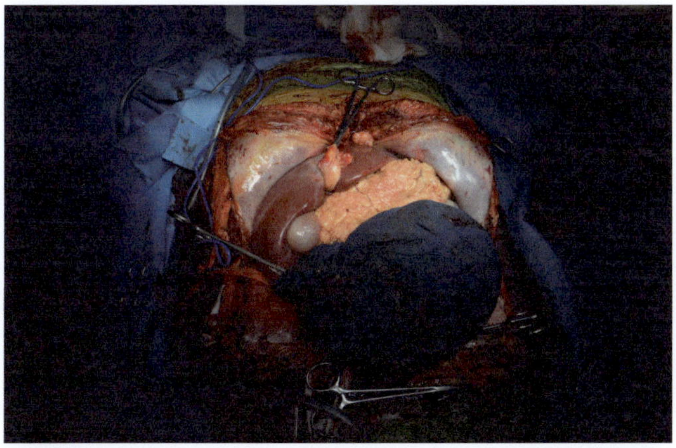

Fig. 1.1 Surgical field of the abdominal cavity during a whole liver graft harvesting in deceased donor

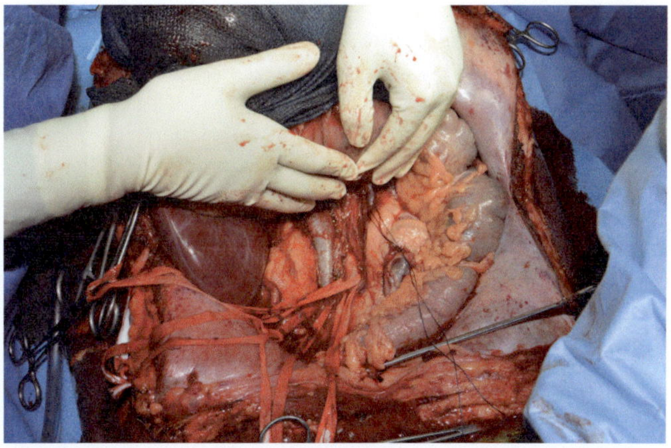

Fig. 1.2 Exposure of the inferior mesenteric vein along the edge of the sigmoid colon lateral to the proximal jejunum

C. Lim et al., *Atlas of Liver Transplantation*, https://doi.org/10.1007/978-3-031-85264-0_1

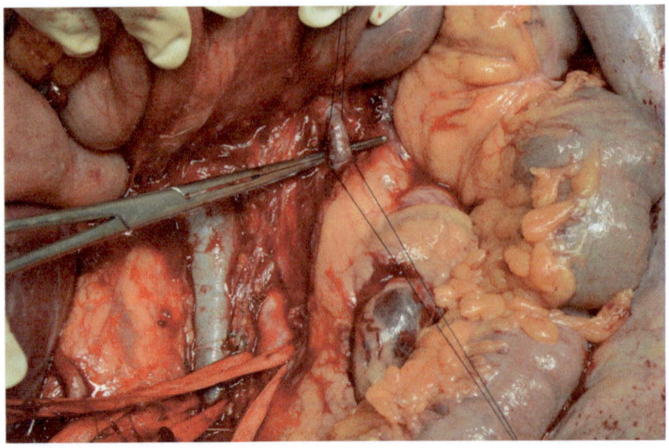

Fig. 1.3 Control of the inferior mesenteric vein

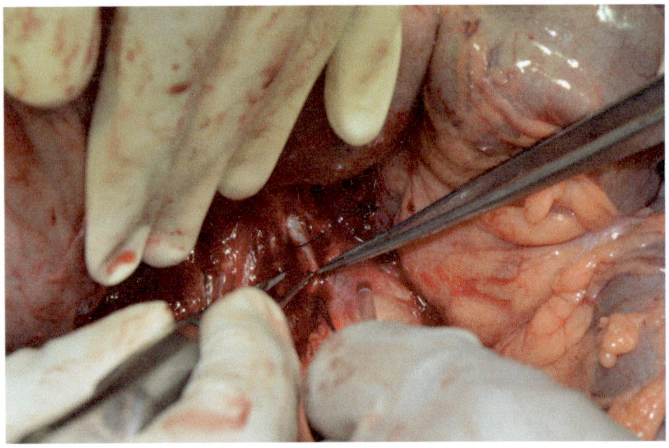

Fig. 1.4 Incision on the anterior wall of the inferior mesenteric vein

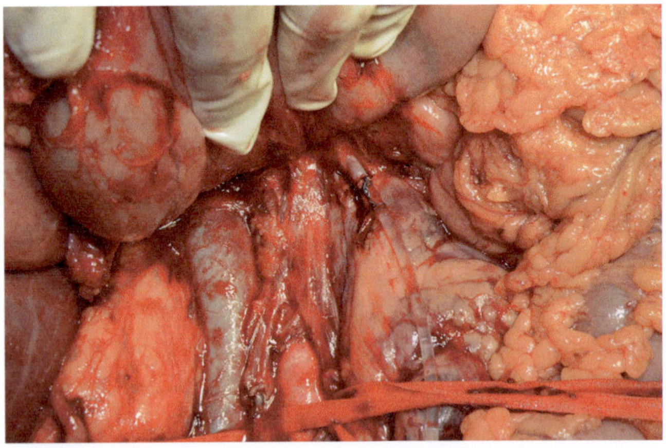

Fig. 1.5 Cannulation of the inferior mesenteric vein for portal cold perfusion

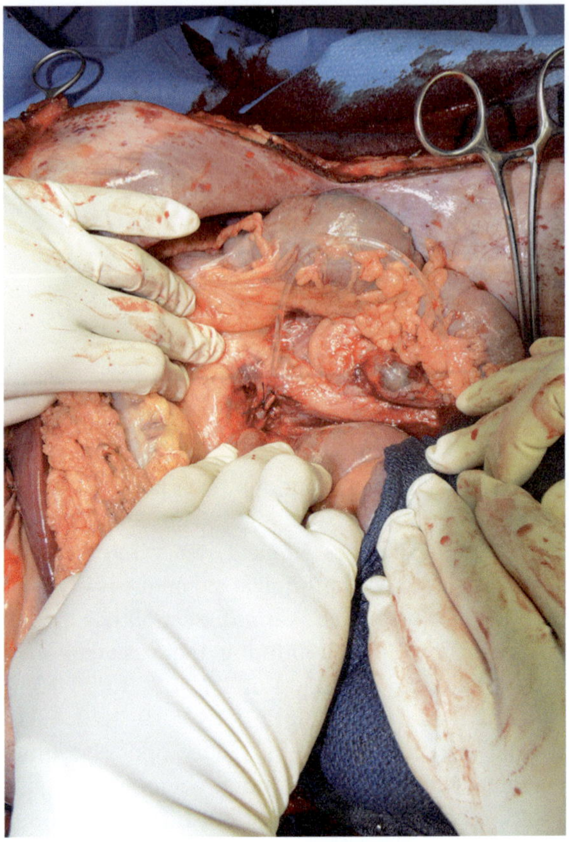

Fig. 1.6 Cannulation of the inferior mesenteric vein

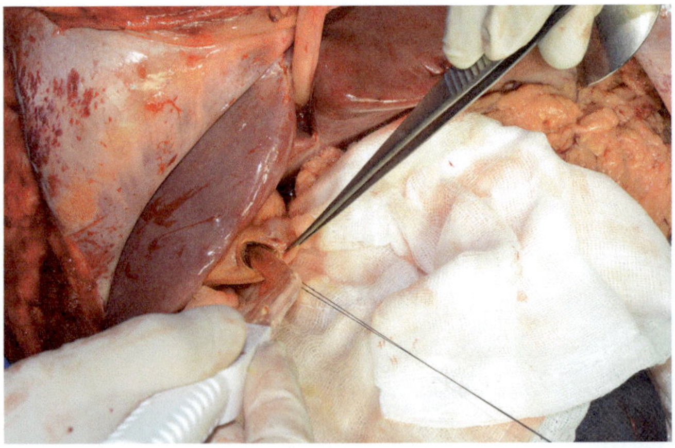

Fig. 1.7 The gallbladder is emptied and flushed with room temperature normal saline

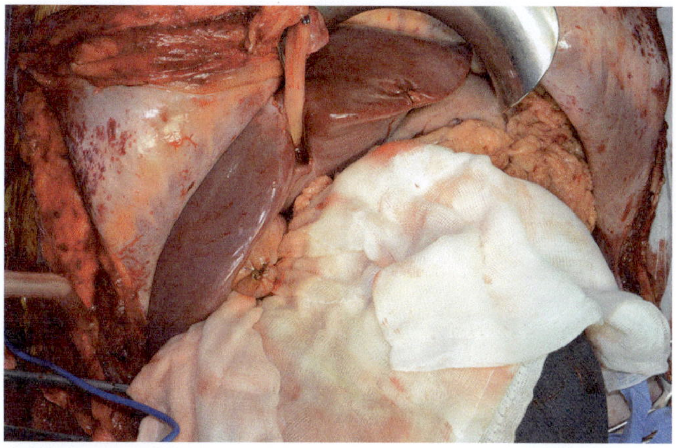

Fig. 1.8 Washing the gallbladder

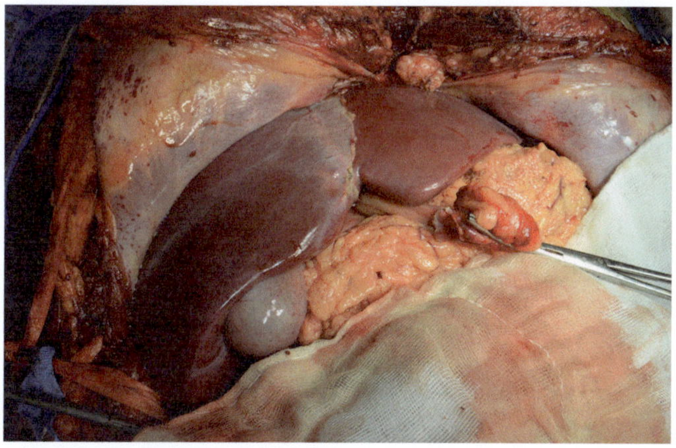

Fig. 1.9 Surgical view of the liver graft

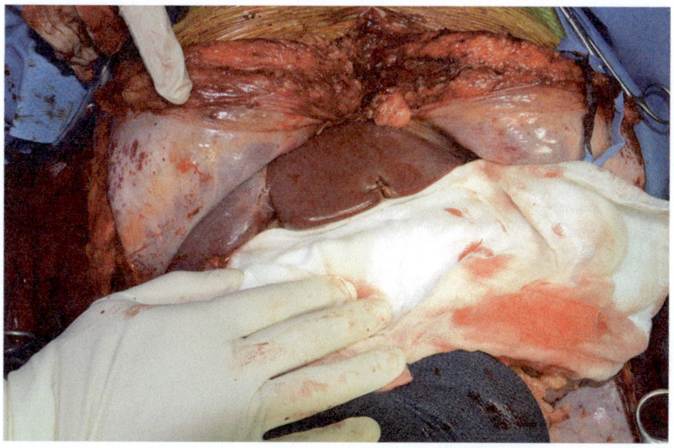

Fig. 1.10 Liver graft biopsy

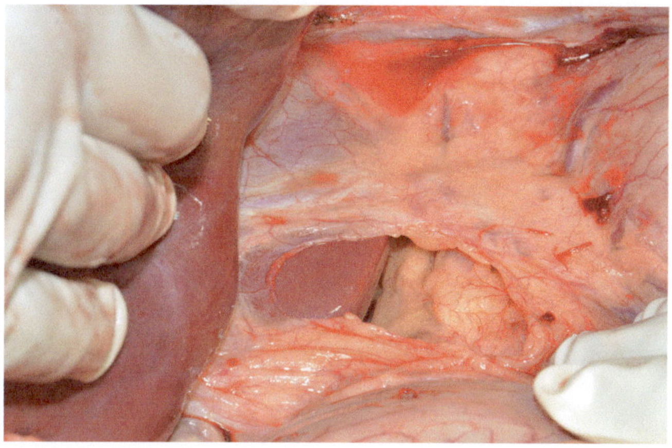

Fig. 1.11 Division of the hepato-gastric ligament confirming the presence of a left accessory hepatic artery arising from the left gastric artery

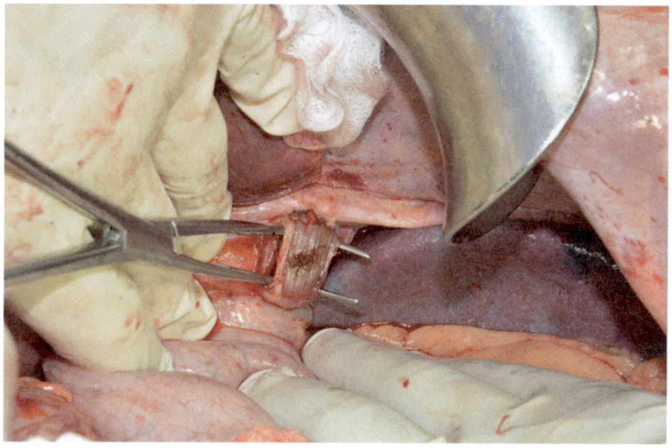

Fig. 1.12 Division of the muscle fibers of the diaphragm and the left accessory hepatic artery is retracted right laterally

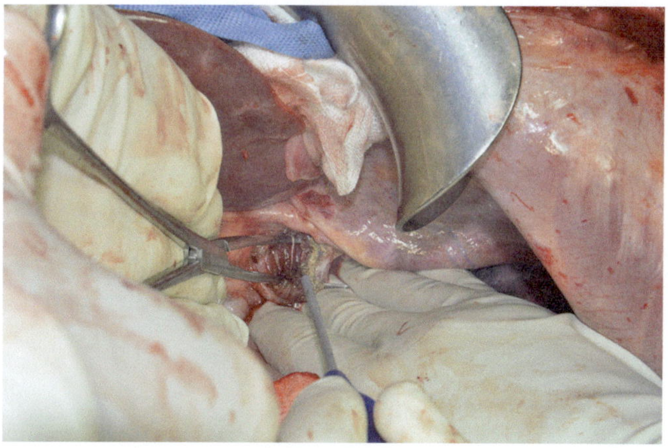

Fig. 1.13 Division of the muscle fibers of the diaphragm

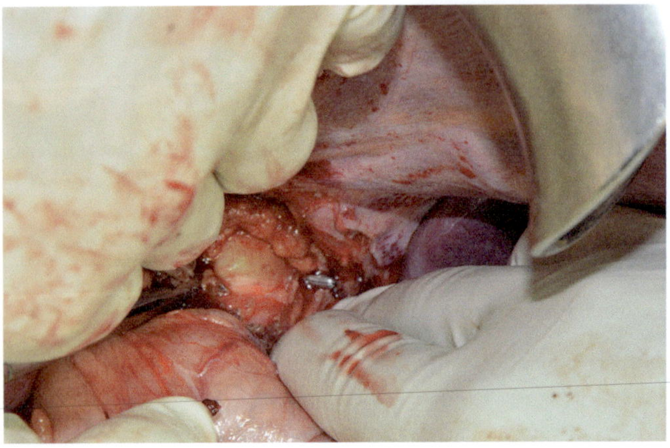

Fig. 1.14 Control of the supraceliac aorta

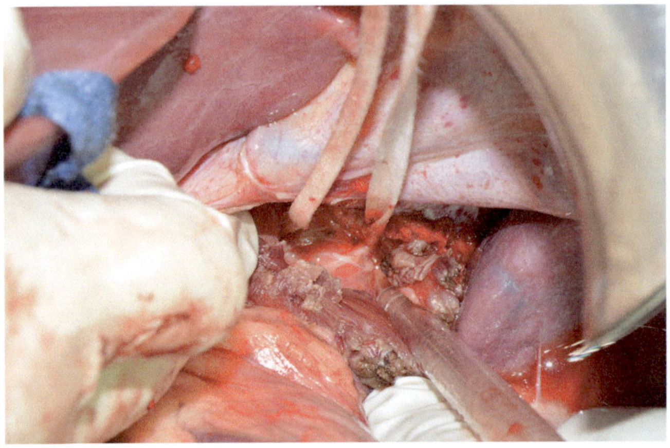

Fig. 1.15 A tape is encircled over this segment of the aorta

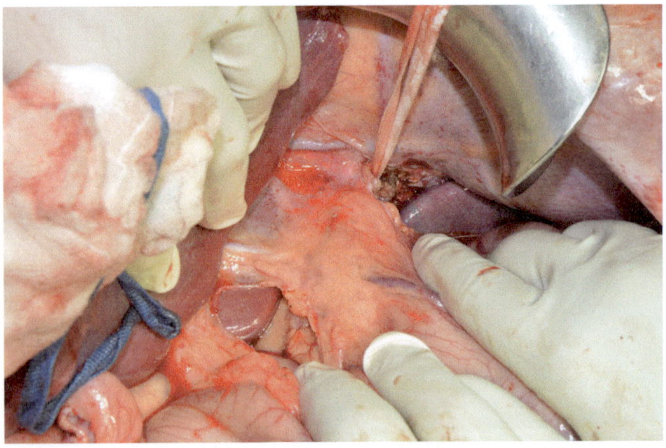

Fig. 1.16 Control of the aorta on the left side of the hepato-gastric ligament to avoid the injury of the left accessory hepatic artery

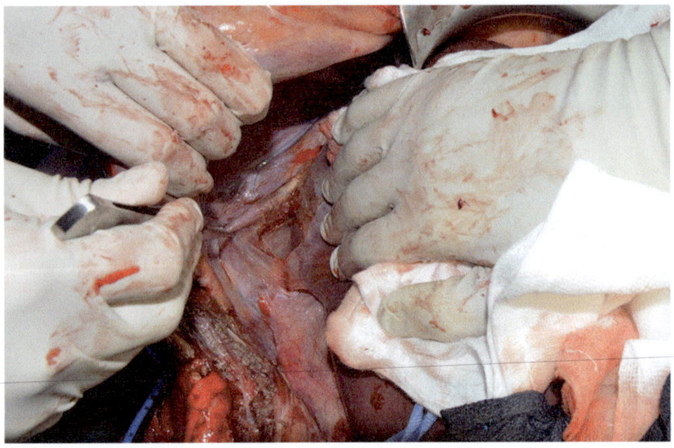

Fig. 1.17 Division of the right triangular ligament to mobilize the right lobe of the liver

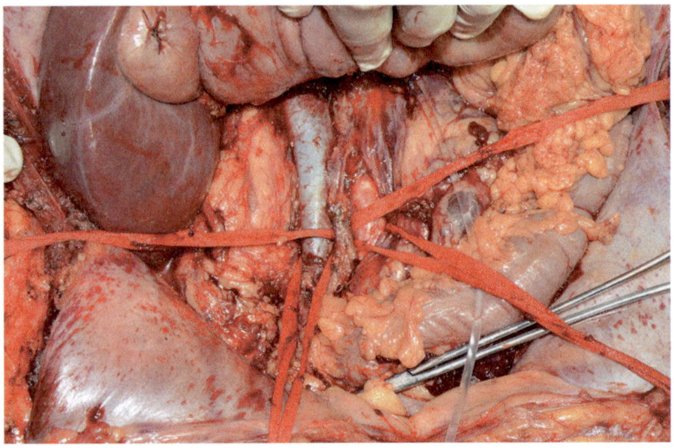

Fig. 1.18 A tape is placed around the distal aortic bifurcation of the common iliac arteries, which is used for ligation of the distal aorta prior to cold perfusion, and another tape is placed around the aorta proximally, which is used for fixing the cannula to the aorta. Two tapes are placed around the inferior vena cava, one for fixing a cannula for adequate perfusion fluid drainage and one for ligation of the confluence of the common iliac veins

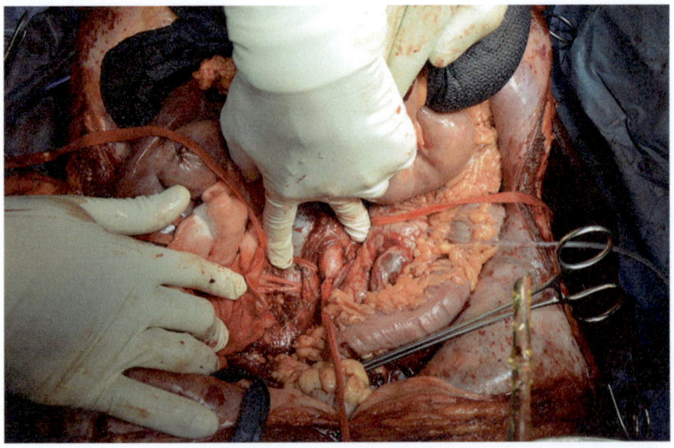

Fig. 1.19 Ligation of the infrarenal aorta

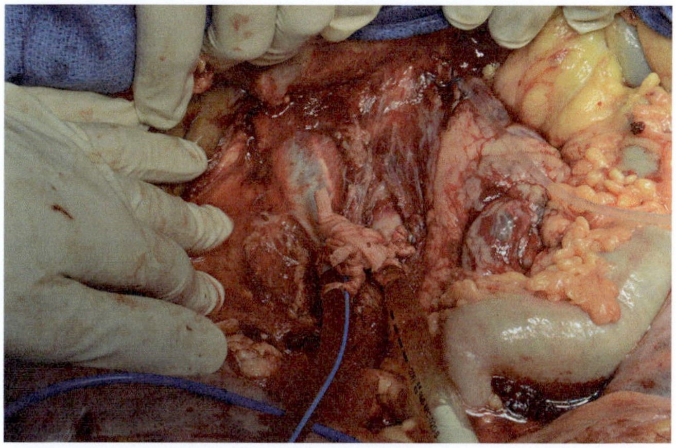

Fig. 1.20 Cannulation of the infrahepatic inferior vena cava (for perfusion drainage) and infrarenal aorta (for cold perfusion)

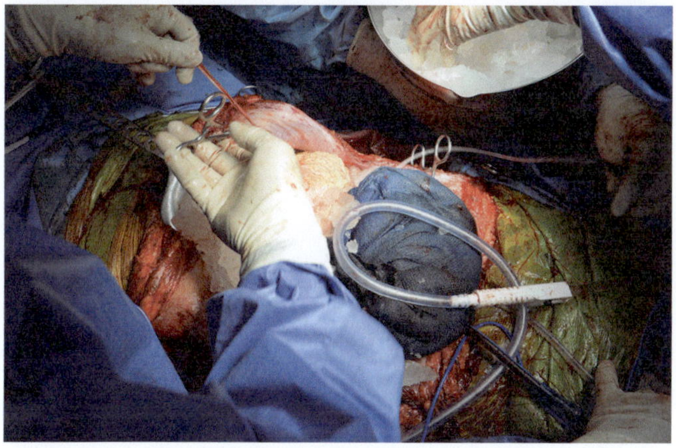

Fig. 1.21 Ligation of the supraceliac aorta

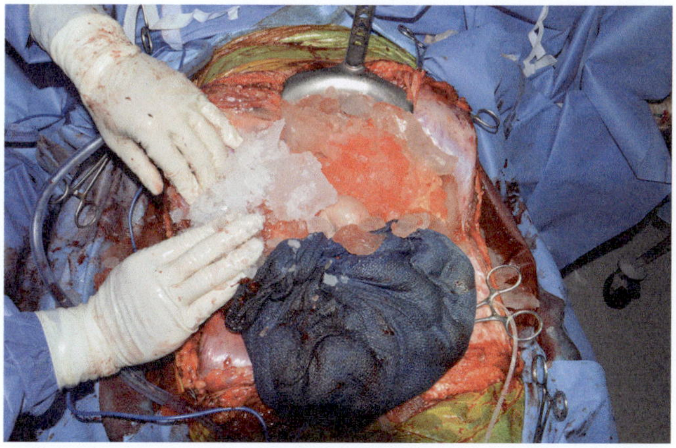

Fig. 1.22 Topical cooling of the liver, pancreas, kidney, and intestine

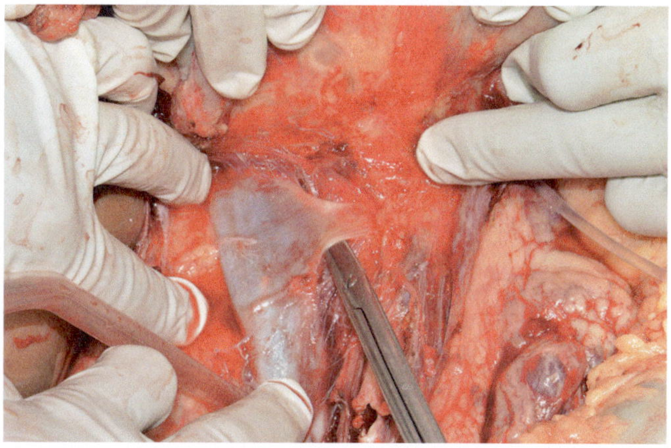

Fig. 1.23 Control of the left renal vein

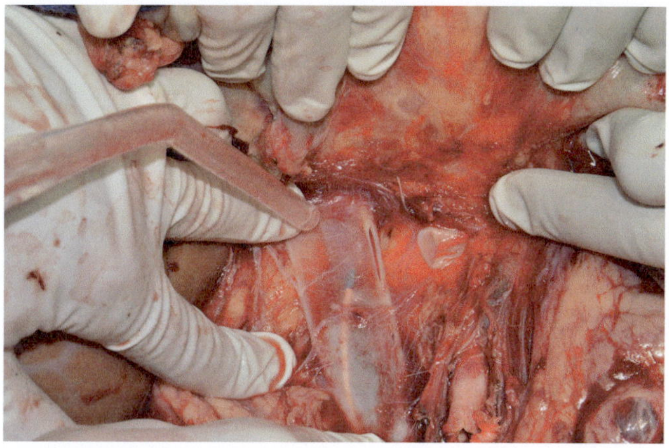

Fig. 1.24 Section of the left renal vein

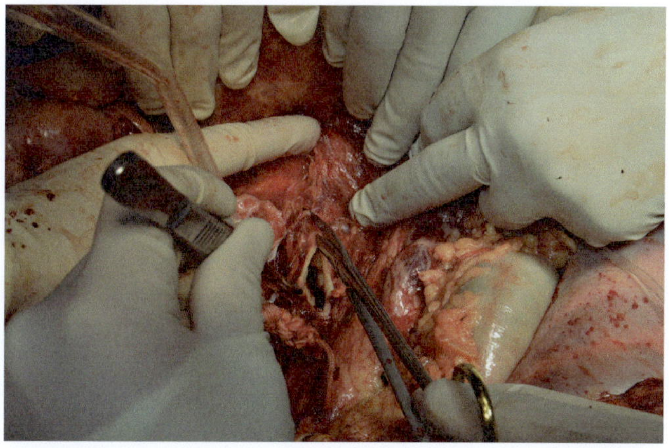

Fig. 1.25 Incision of the anterior wall of the aorta just below the level of the renal artery

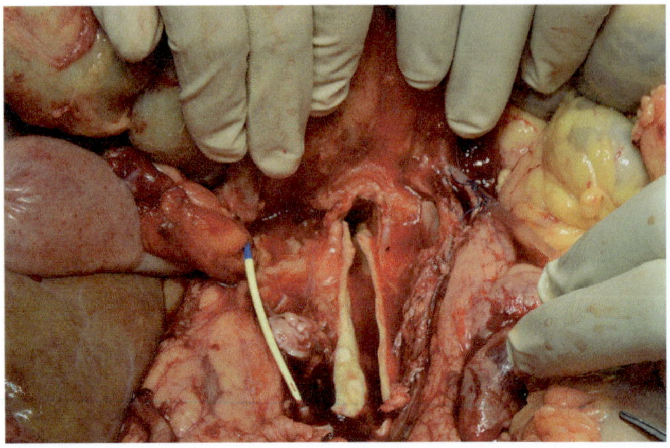

Fig. 1.26 Incision of the anterior wall of the aorta

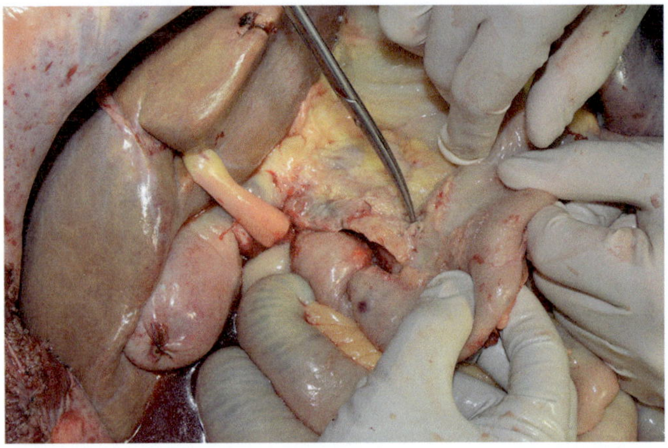

Fig. 1.27 Dissection of the common bile duct at the level to the upper margin of the duodenum

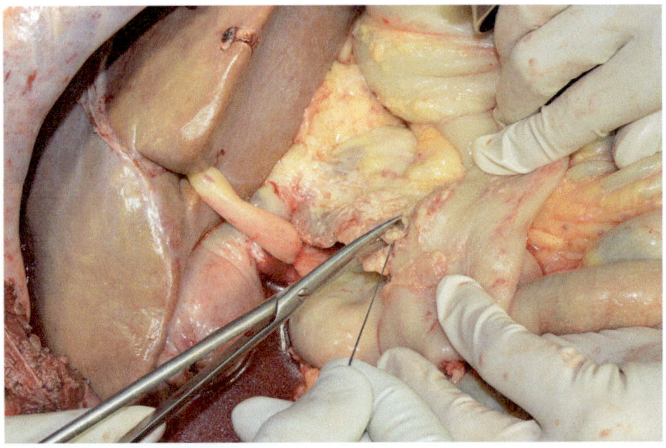

Fig. 1.28 Transection of the common bile duct

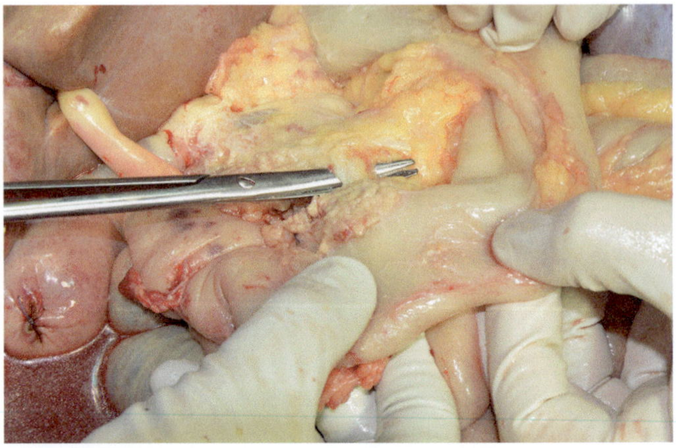

Fig. 1.29 Dissection of the gastroduodenal artery

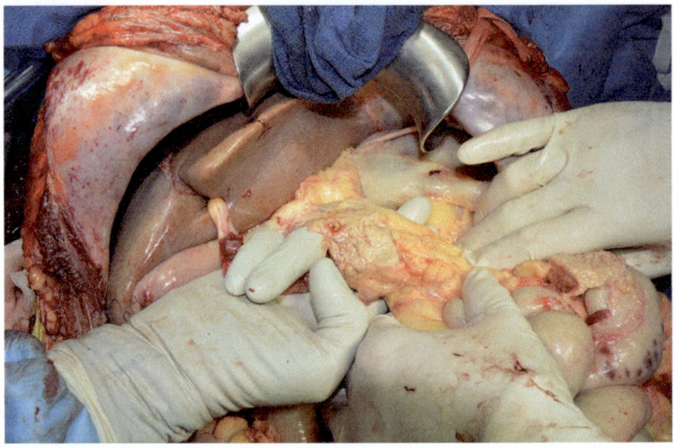

Fig. 1.30 Dissection of the head of the pancreas from the duodenum (the en-bloc technique includes the pancreas head)

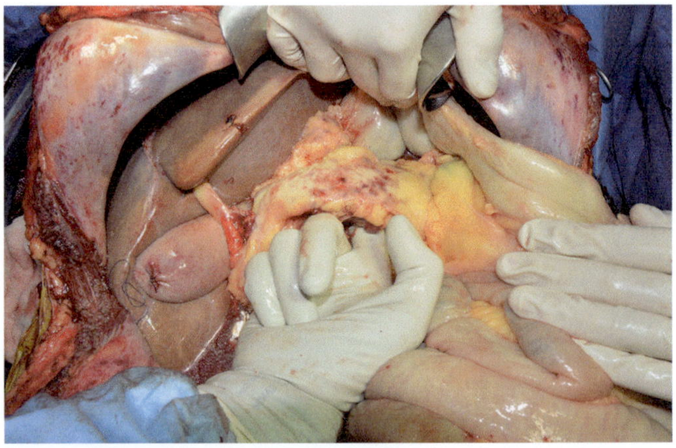

Fig. 1.31 Control of the pancreas isthmus

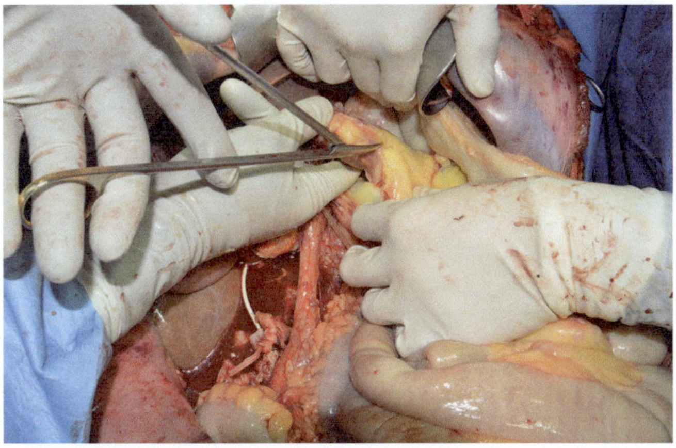

Fig. 1.32 Transection of the pancreas isthmus

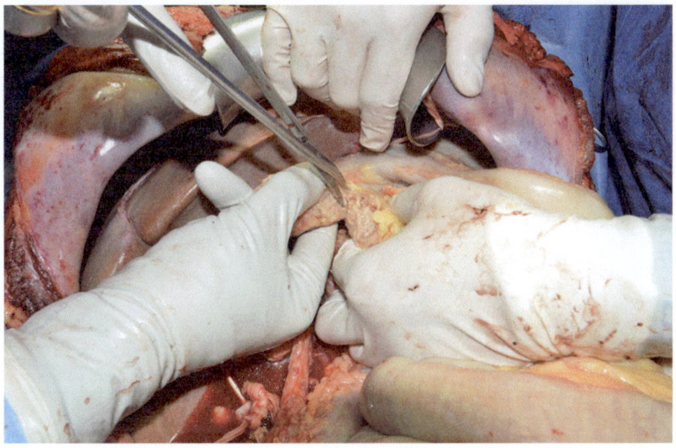

Fig. 1.33 Transection of the pancreas isthmus

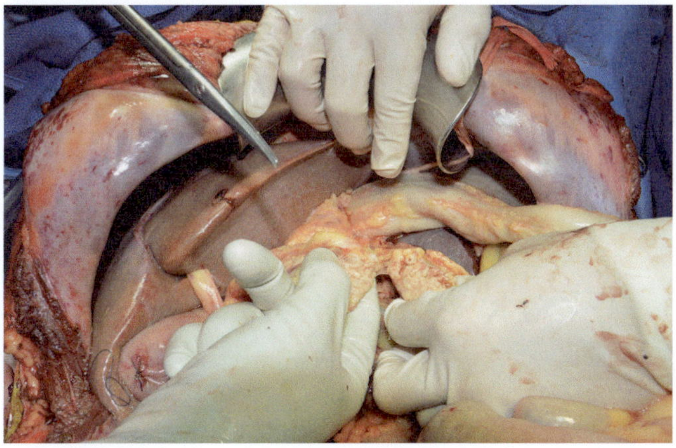

Fig. 1.34 Transection of the pancreas isthmus

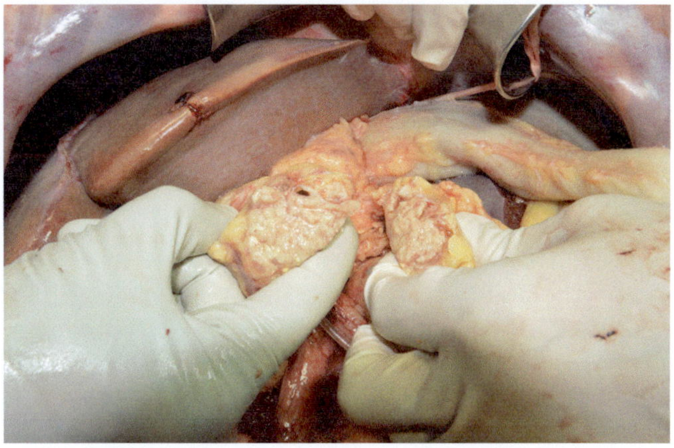

Fig. 1.35 Transection of the pancreas isthmus

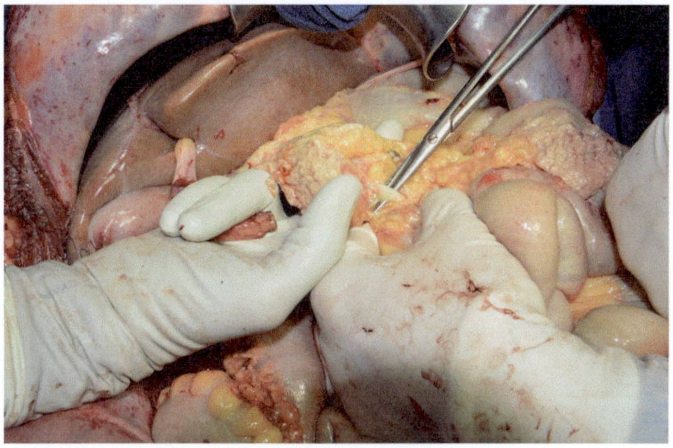

Fig. 1.36 Division of the superior mesenteric artery at the lower part of the pancreas

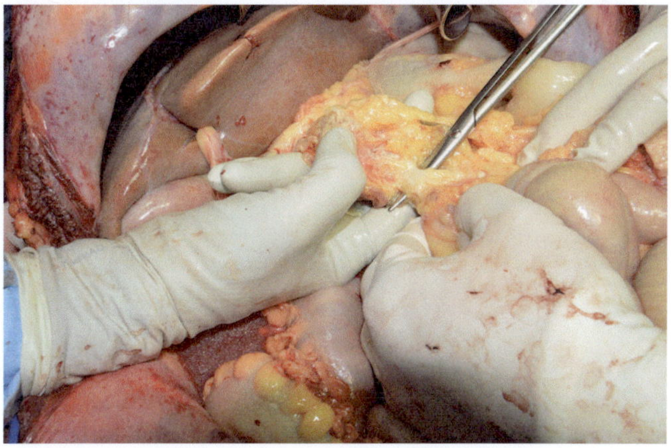

Fig. 1.37 Division of the superior mesenteric vein at the lower part of the pancreas

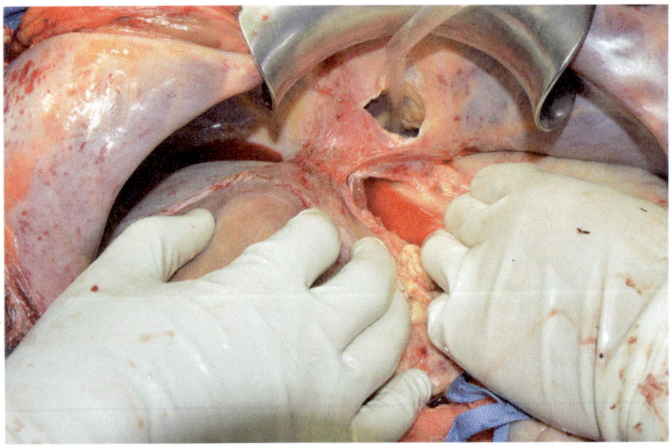

Fig. 1.38 Incision of the diaphragm

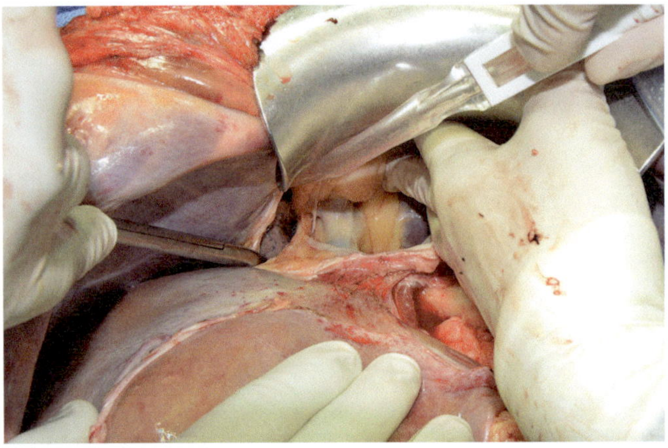

Fig. 1.39 Division of the inferior vena cava just below the right atrium

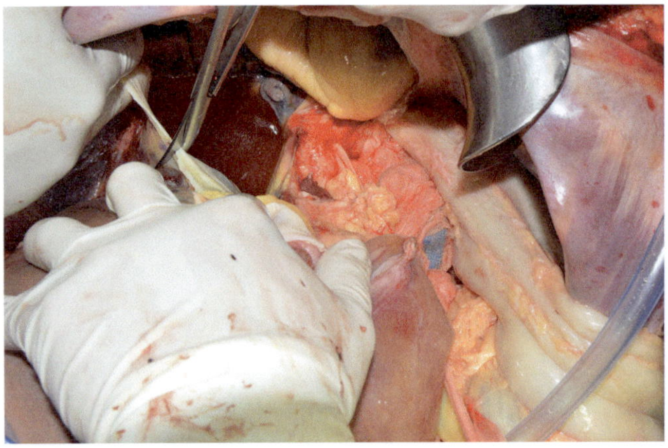

Fig. 1.40 Transection of the diaphragm

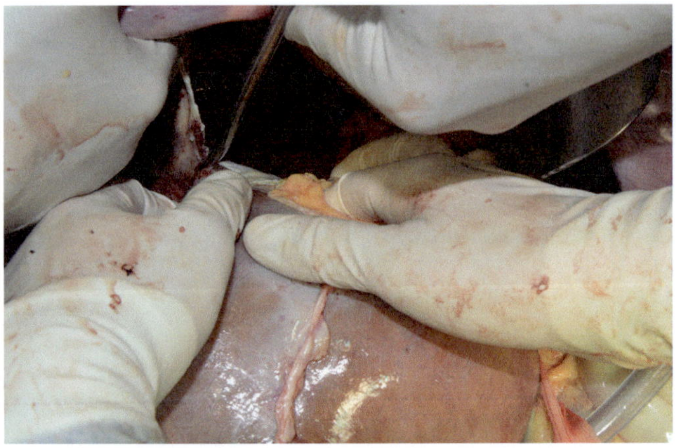

Fig. 1.41 Transection of the diaphragm

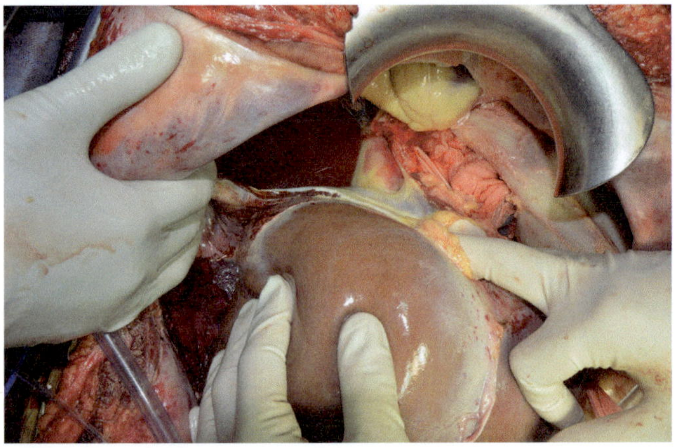

Fig. 1.42 Transection of the diaphragm

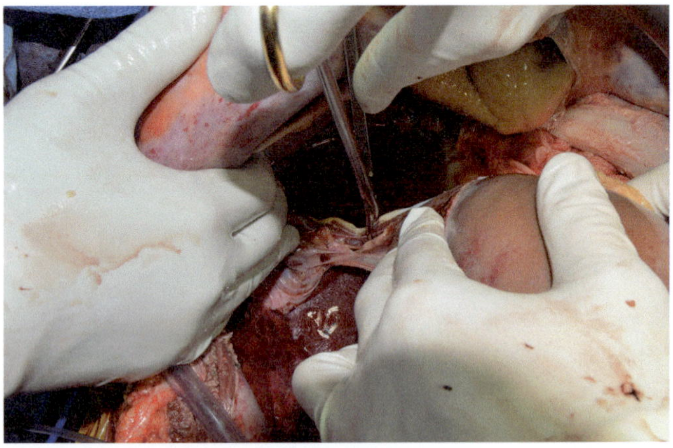

Fig. 1.43 Transection of the diaphragm

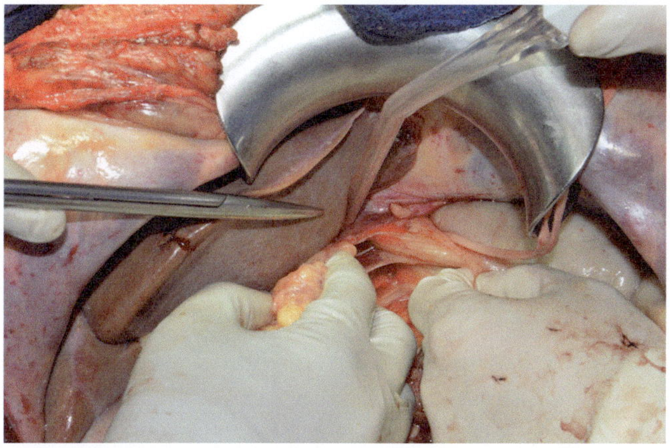

Fig. 1.44 Completion of the hepato-gastric ligament division to mobilize the left lateral section of the liver

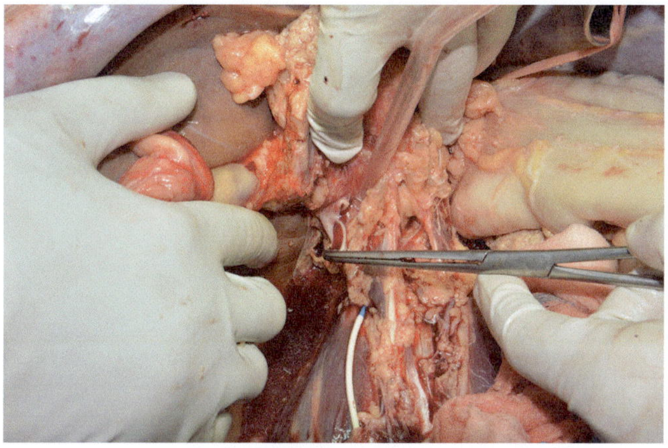

Fig. 1.45 Dissection of the posterior part of the infrahepatic inferior vena cava

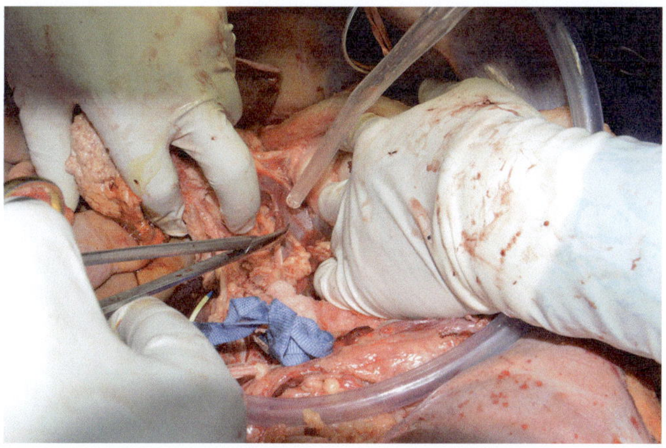

Fig. 1.46 Section of the muscular fibers of the diaphragm to expose the left side of the aorta

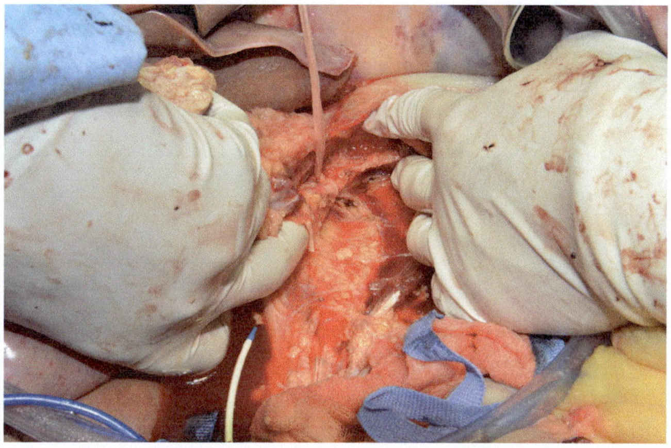

Fig. 1.47 Transection of the muscular fibers of the diaphragm to expose the left part of the aorta using the finger of the surgeon to avoid injury

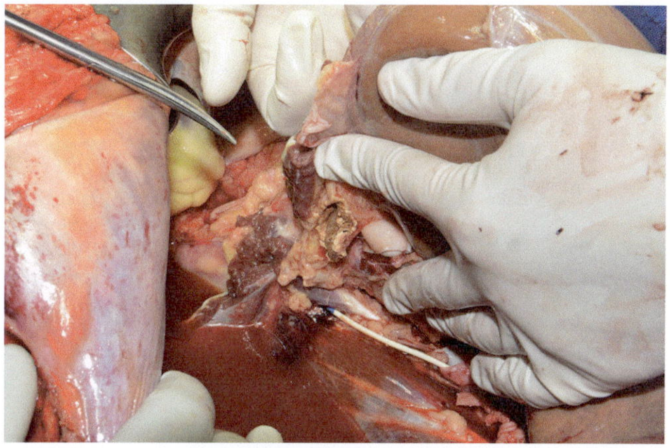

Fig. 1.48 Transection of the muscular fibers of the diaphragm to expose the right part of the inferior vena cava using the finger of the surgeon to avoid injury

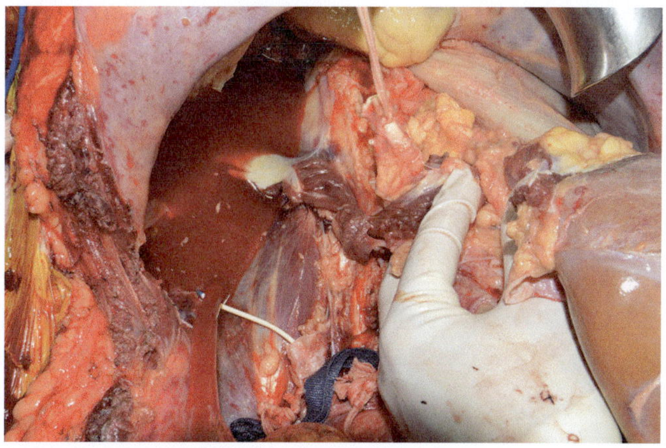

Fig. 1.49 Transection of the muscular fibers of the diaphragm to expose the right part of the aorta using the finger of the surgeon before achieving total hepatectomy

Reference

1. Van Thiel DH, Schade RR, Hakala TR, Starzl TE, Denny D. Liver procurement for orthotopic transplantation: an analysis of the Pittsburgh experience. Hepatology. 1984;4(1 Suppl):66S–71S. https://doi.org/10.1002/hep.1840040718.

2 Back-Table Procedure of a Whole Liver Graft for the Piggyback Technique

The back-table procedure, a major step in orthotopic liver transplantation, constitutes the final stage of liver procurement and is usually performed in the recipient operating room.

The back-table preparation includes the following six steps: It begins with the dissection of the inferior vena cava, the portal vein, the superior mesenteric artery, and the celiac trunk, continues with the common hepatic artery, and concludes with the bile duct. The supra- and infrahepatic inferior vena cava are then closed using a vascular stapler or with Prolene continuous sutures. Finally, the posterior wall of the retrohepatic inferior vena cava is opened for the piggyback technique (Figs. 2.1, 2.2, 2.3, 2.4, 2.5, 2.6, 2.7, 2.8, 2.9, 2.10, 2.11, 2.12, 2.13, 2.14, 2.15, 2.16, 2.17, 2.18, 2.19, 2.20, 2.21, 2.22, 2.23, 2.24, 2.25, 2.26, 2.27, 2.28, 2.29, 2.30, 2.31, 2.32, and 2.33).

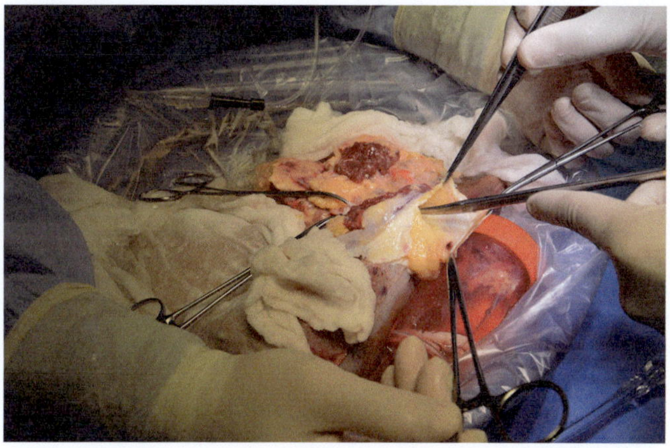

Fig. 2.1 Preparation of the donor inferior vena cava

C. Lim et al., *Atlas of Liver Transplantation*, https://doi.org/10.1007/978-3-031-85264-0_2

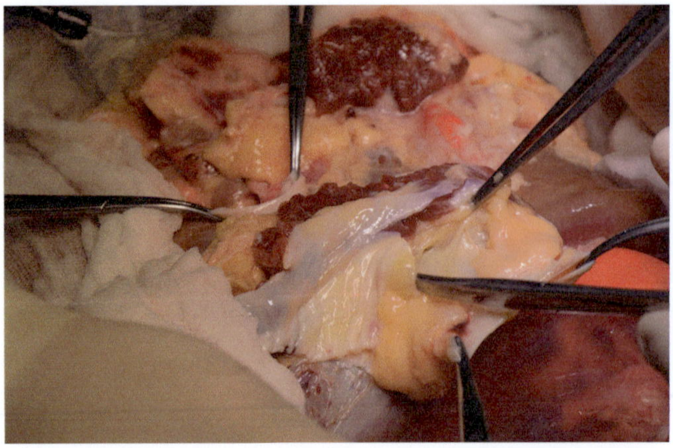

Fig. 2.2 Dissection of the posterior aspect of the suprahepatic inferior vena cava

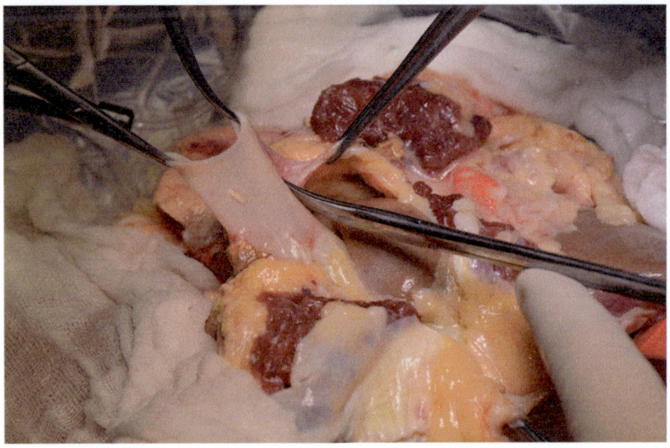

Fig. 2.3 Dissection of the posterior aspect of the infrahepatic inferior vena cava

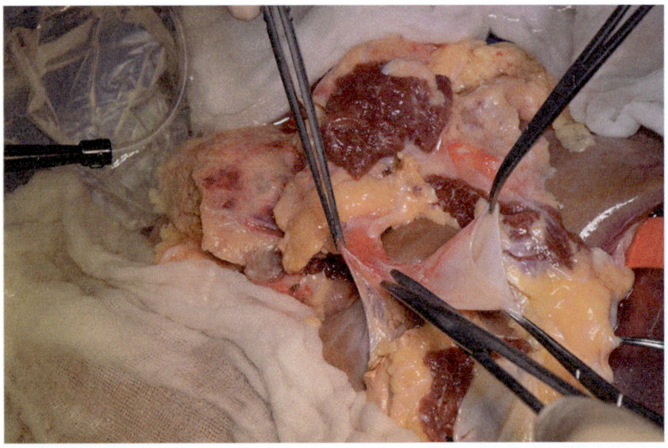

Fig. 2.4 Dissection of the anterior aspect of the infrahepatic inferior vena cava

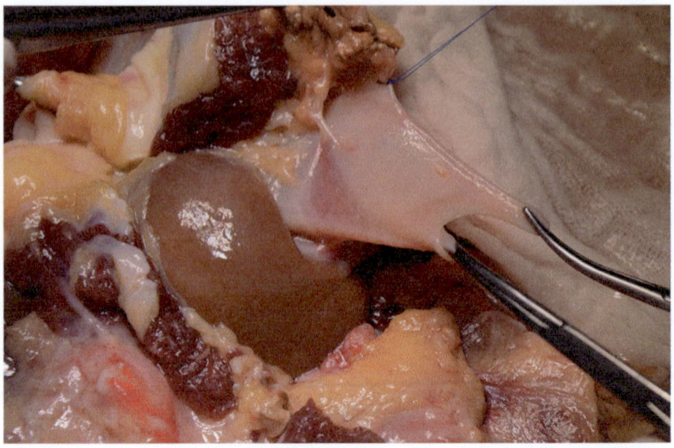

Fig. 2.5 Dissection of the posterior aspect of the suprahepatic inferior vena cava with ligation of a small phrenic vein

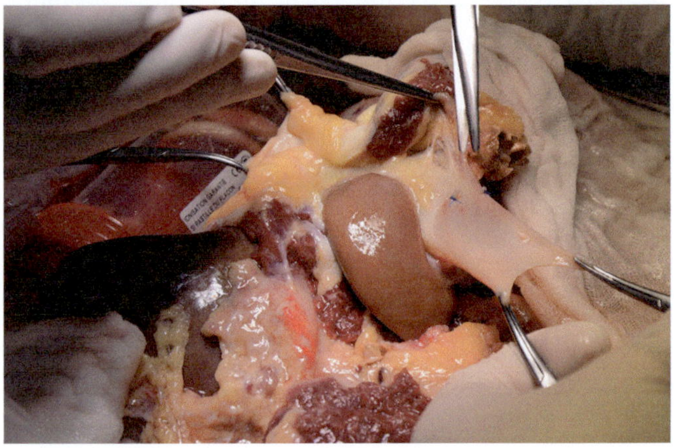

Fig. 2.6 Dissection of the right part of posterior aspect of the retrohepatic inferior vena cava

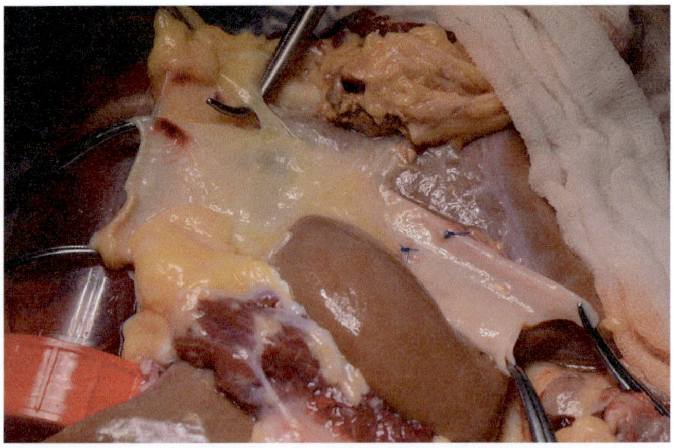

Fig. 2.7 Dissection of the right aspect of the retrohepatic inferior vena cava with control of the right adrenal vein

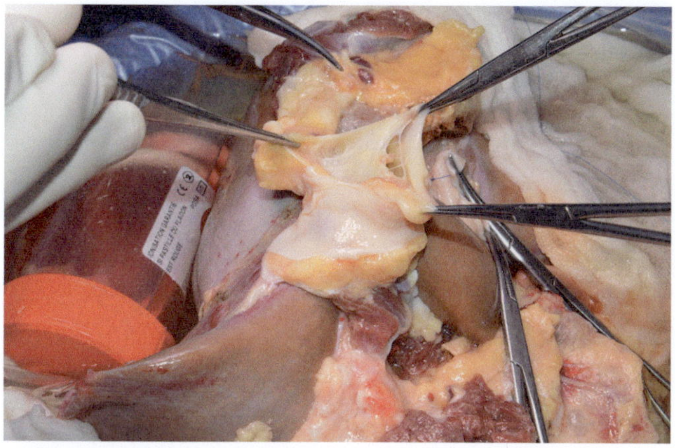

Fig. 2.8 Dissection of the anterior aspect of the suprahepatic inferior vena cava

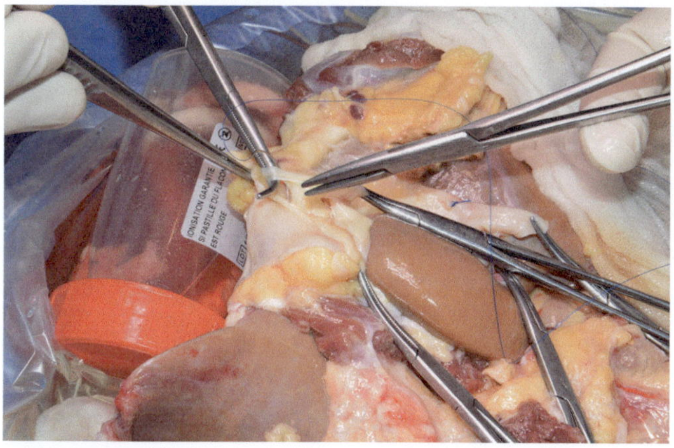

Fig. 2.9 Dissection of the anterior aspect of the suprahepatic inferior vena cava with control of a phrenic vein

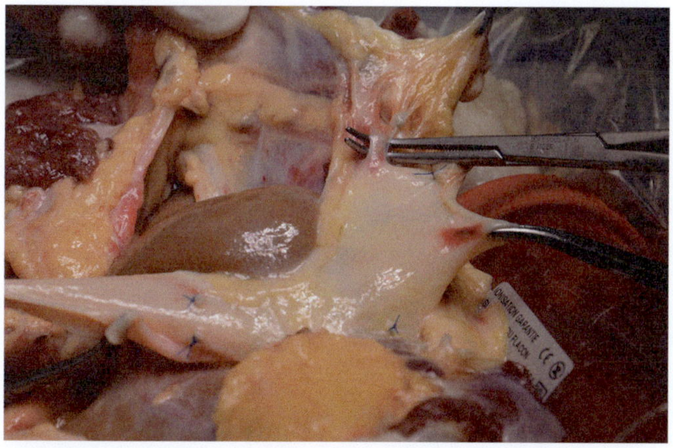

Fig. 2.10 Dissection of the anterior aspect of the suprahepatic inferior vena cava with control of another phrenic vein

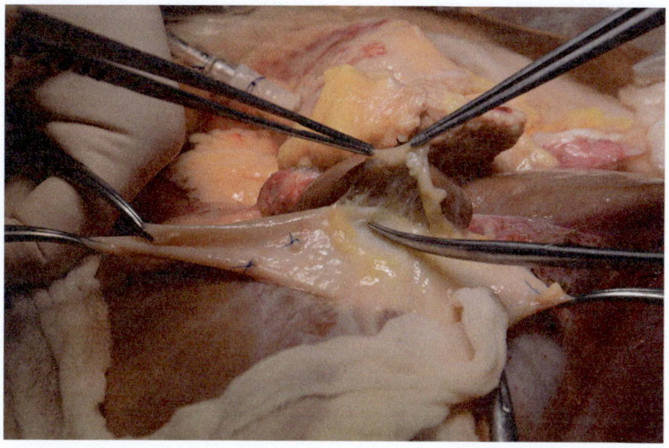

Fig. 2.11 Division of the ligament of the inferior vena cava and mobilization of the caudate lobe to expose the retrohepatic inferior vena cava

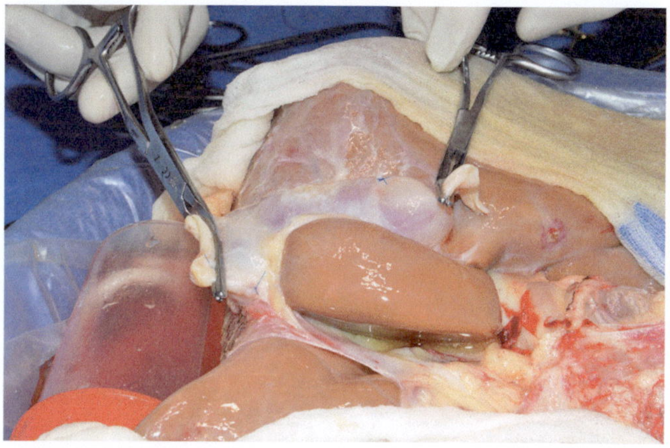

Fig. 2.12 Clamping of the supra- and infrahepatic inferior vena cava to identify any iatrogenic injury to the inferior vena cava

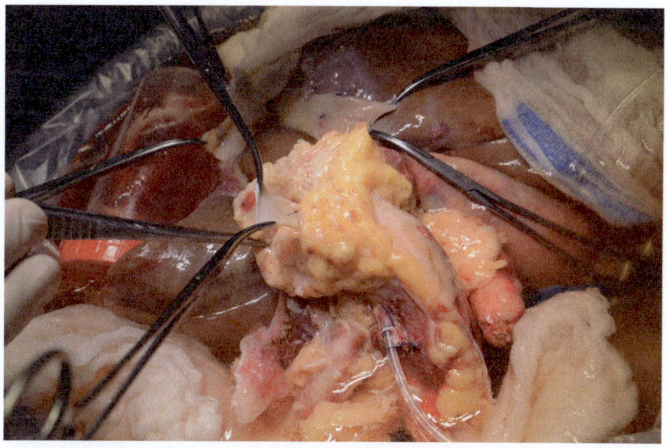

Fig. 2.13 Dissection of the anterior aspect of the portal vein from the posterior part of the pancreas

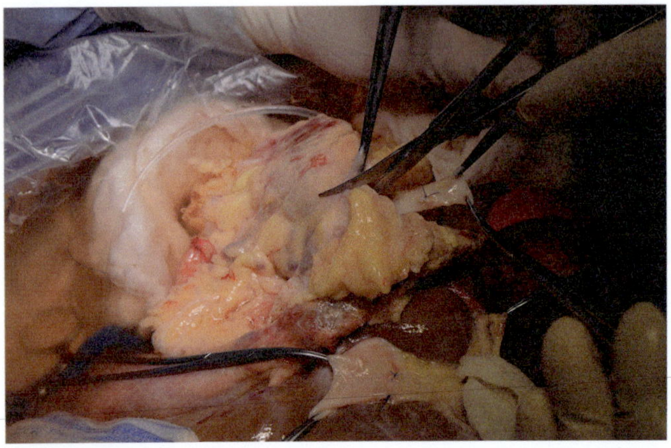

Fig. 2.14 Transection of the pancreas

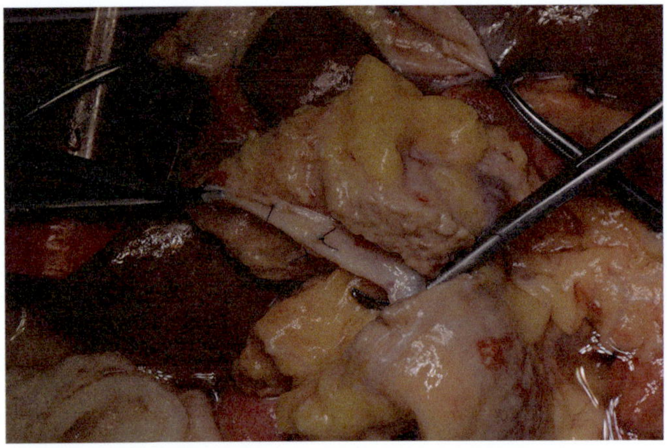

Fig. 2.15 Control of the splenic vein

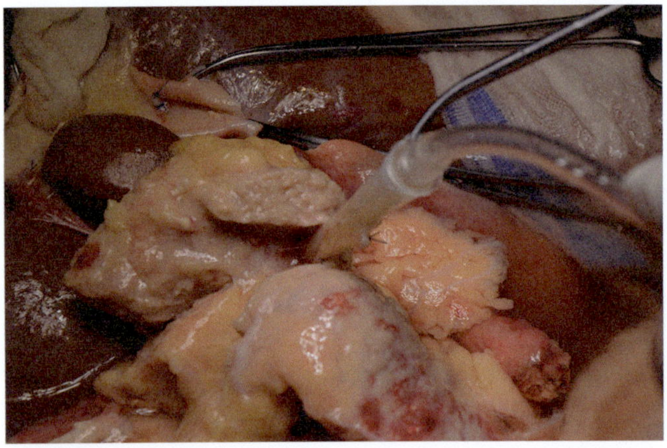

Fig. 2.16 Transection of the pancreas showing the portal vein

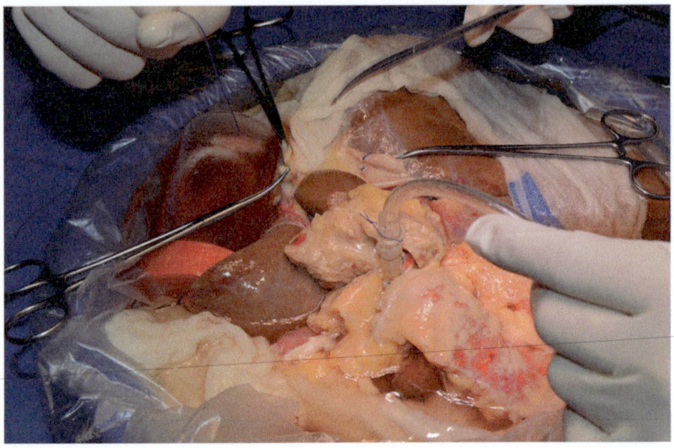

Fig. 2.17 The portal vein is cannulated for portal cold perfusion of the graft

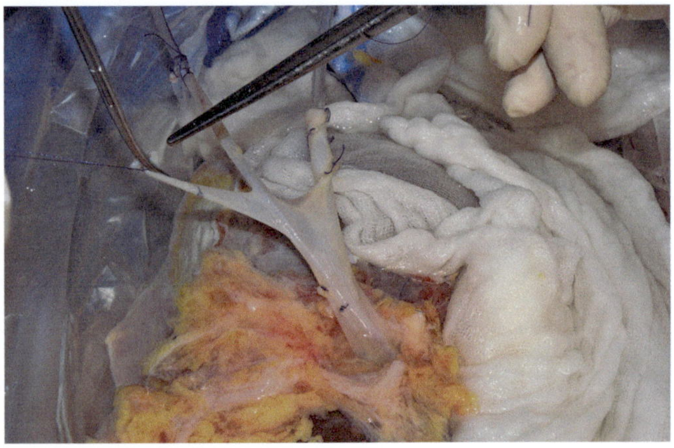

Fig. 2.18 Surgical view of the mesentericoportal axis after removing the pancreas

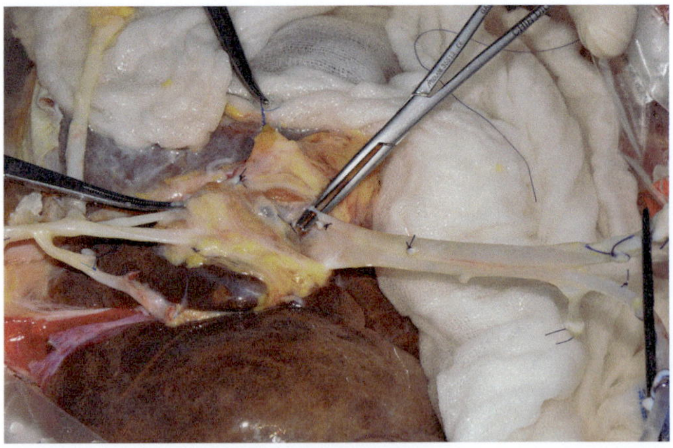

Fig. 2.19 Looking for the portal bifurcation. (Note: In that case, the hepatic artery has been dissected first)

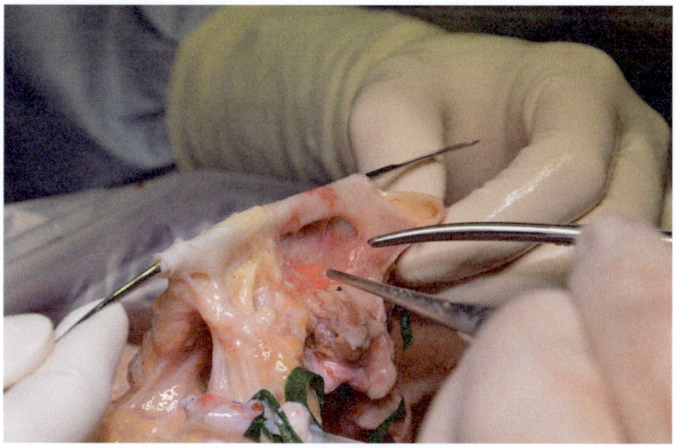

Fig. 2.20 Dissection of the posterior aspect of the superior mesenteric artery

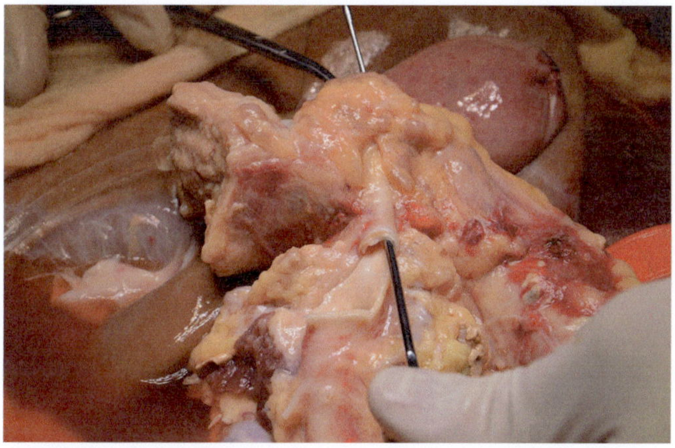

Fig. 2.21 Dissection of the posterior aspect of the superior mesenteric artery

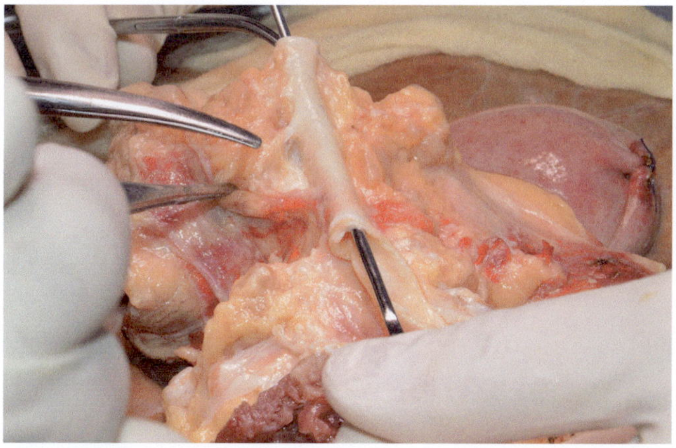

Fig. 2.22 Dissection of the superior mesenteric artery to detect an accessory right hepatic artery

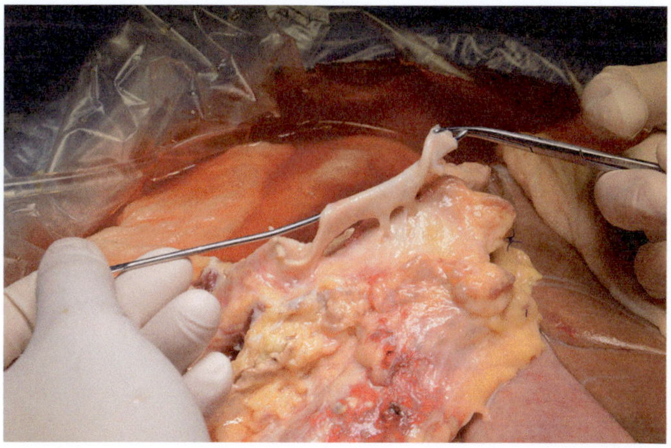

Fig. 2.23 Dissection of the anterior aspect of the superior mesenteric artery showing some jejunal and pancreatic arteries

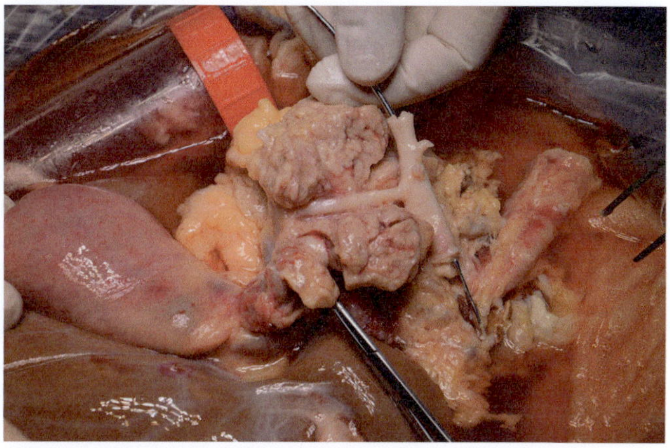

Fig. 2.24 Dissection of the arterial inflow from the aortic patch, cleaning off the celiac plexus and fatty tissue enveloping the arteries

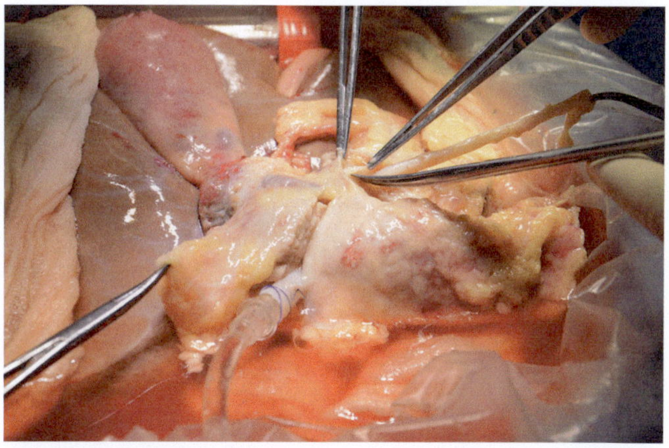

Fig. 2.25 Dissection of the splenic artery at the superior part of the pancreas to the level of the gastroduodenal artery (mosquito forceps is applied to the corner of the gastroduodenal artery)

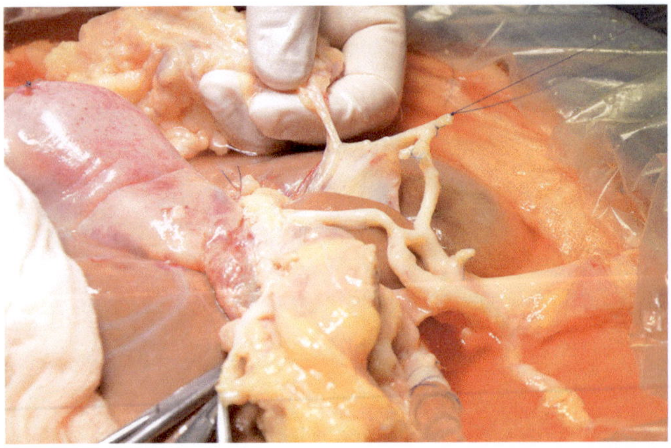

Fig. 2.26 Dissection of the left gastric artery including an accessory left hepatic artery

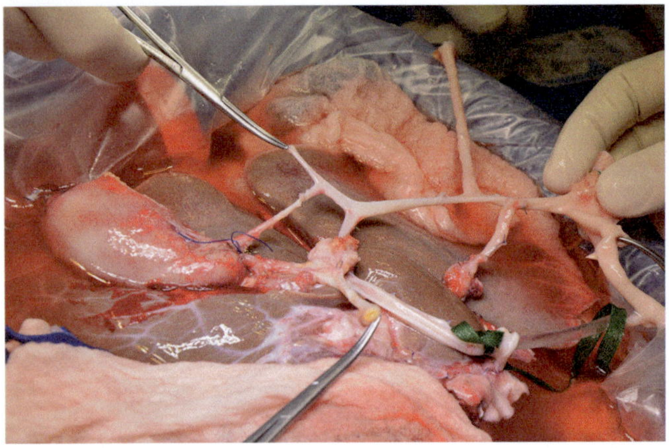

Fig. 2.27 Liver graft with a common hepatic artery (mosquito forceps is applied to the corner of the gastroduodenal artery)

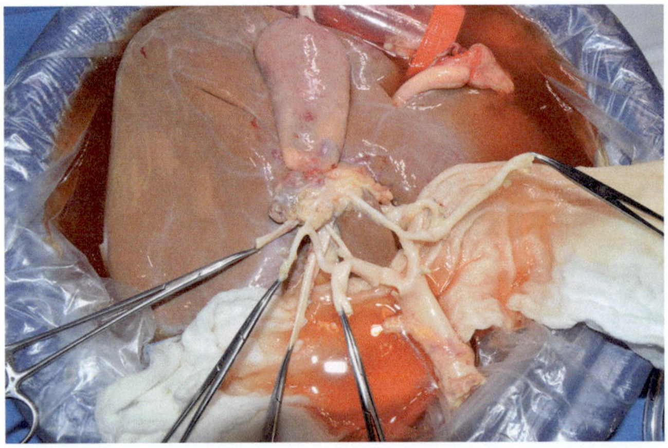

Fig. 2.28 Liver graft with two arteries: a common hepatic artery and a replaced right hepatic artery arising from the superior mesenteric artery

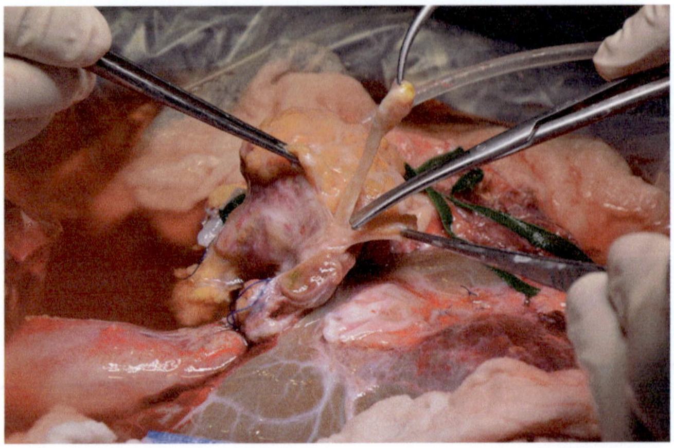

Fig. 2.29 Dissection of the bile duct at the level of the pancreas

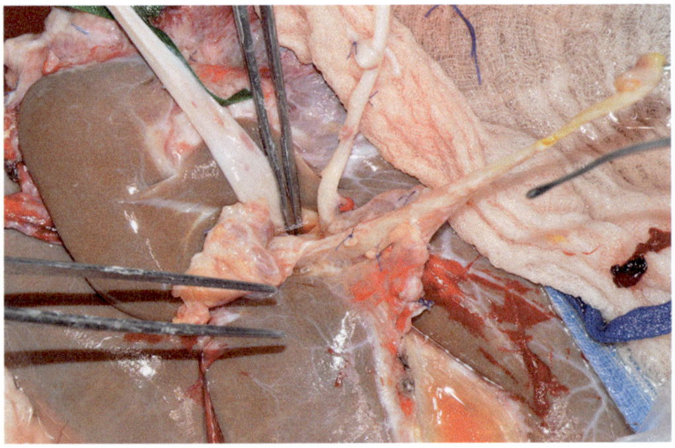

Fig. 2.30 Dissection of the bile duct above the pancreas

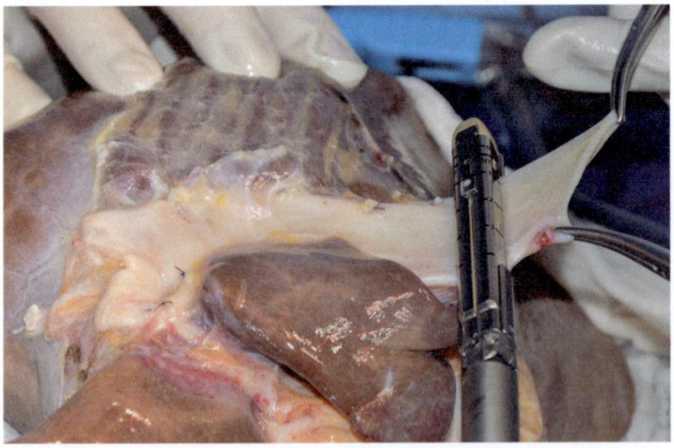

Fig. 2.31 Closure of the infrahepatic inferior vena cava

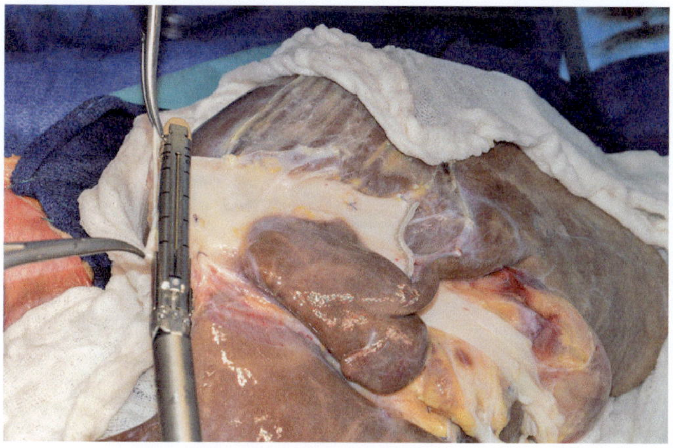

Fig. 2.32 Closure of the suprahepatic inferior vena cava

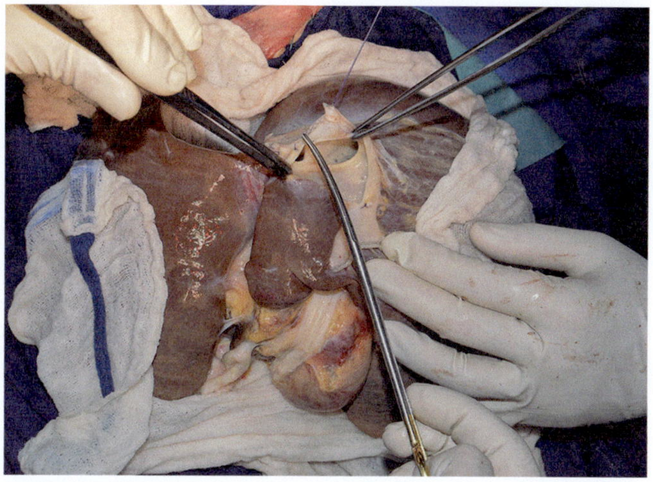

Fig. 2.33 Incision of the posterior wall of the inferior vena cava for piggyback technique

3 Piggyback Total Hepatectomy

The standard technical procedure of a piggyback total hepatectomy includes preservation of the native inferior vena cava [1–7] and a temporary end-to-side portocaval shunt, according to the surgeon's preference and the liver transplantation scenario. During the recipient total hepatectomy, each element of the hepatic pedicle (hepatic artery, bile duct, and portal vein) is dissected, ligated, and transected. The retrohepatic inferior vena cava is then dissected, and the native liver is progressively separated from the native inferior vena cava (Figs. 3.1, 3.2, 3.3, 3.4, 3.5, 3.6, 3.7, 3.8, 3.9, 3.10, 3.11, 3.12, 3.13, 3.14, 3.15, 3.16, 3.17, 3.18, 3.19, 3.20, 3.21, 3.22, 3.23, 3.24, 3.25, 3.26, 3.27, 3.28, 3.29, 3.30, 3.31, 3.32, 3.33, 3.34, 3.35, 3.36, 3.37, 3.38, 3.39, 3.40, and 3.41).

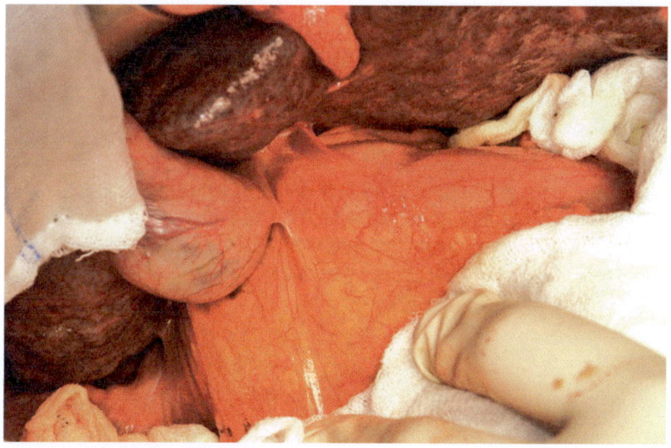

Fig. 3.1 Exposing the hepatic pedicle

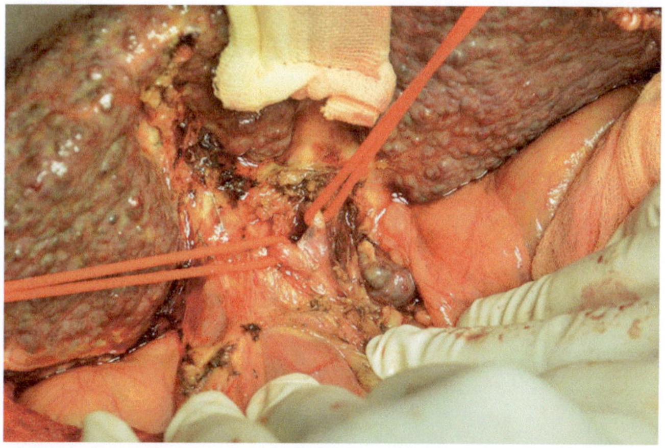

Fig. 3.2 Control of the left branch of the hepatic artery and the arterial branch of segment IV

C. Lim et al., *Atlas of Liver Transplantation*, https://doi.org/10.1007/978-3-031-85264-0_3

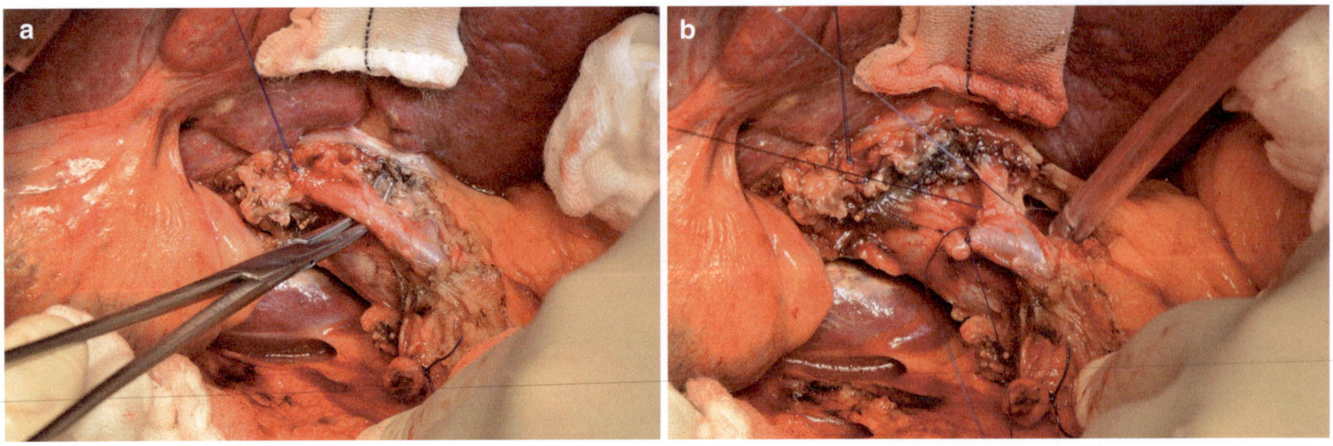

Fig. 3.3 Dissecting the proper hepatic artery. (**a**) Isolating the right branch of the hepatic artery. (**b**) Isolating the left branch of the hepatic artery after ligation and division of the right branch of the hepatic artery

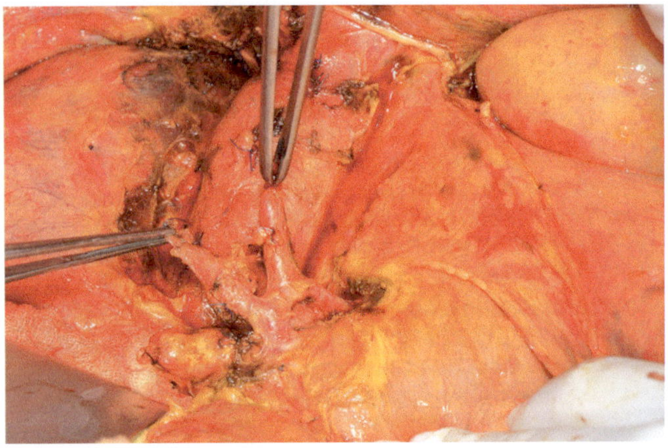

Fig. 3.4 The right and left branches of the hepatic artery have been ligated and divided

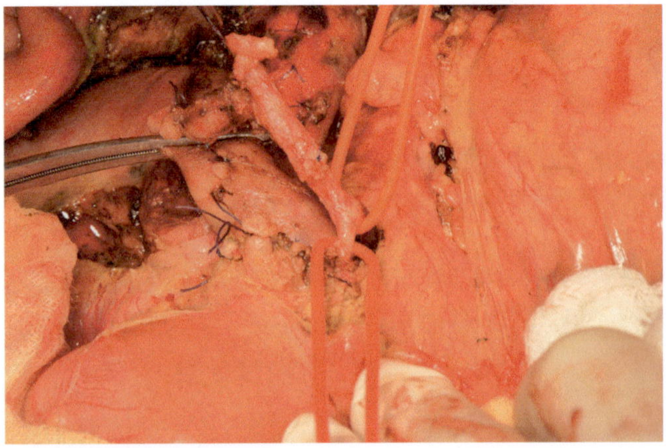

Fig. 3.5 The common hepatic artery and gastroduodenal artery have been isolated and taped

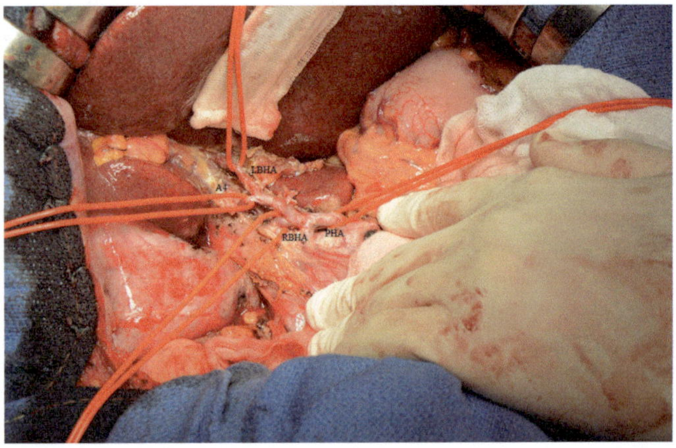

Fig. 3.6 The right (RBHA) and left (LBHA) branches of the hepatic artery, the arterial branch of segment IV (A4), and the proper hepatic artery (PHA) have been isolated and taped

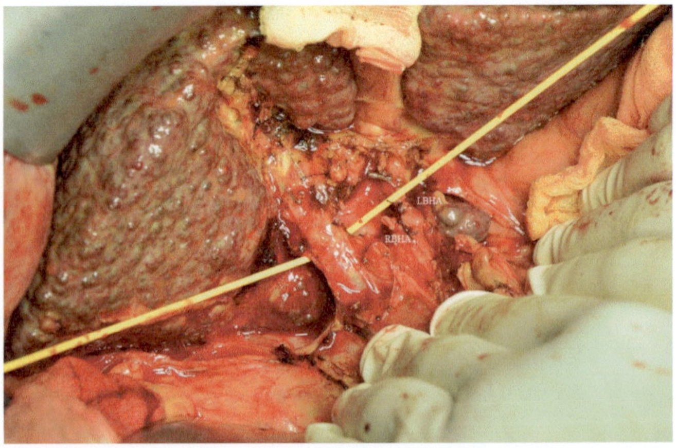

Fig. 3.7 After division of the left (LBHA) and right (RBHA) branches of the hepatic artery, the common bile duct has been isolated and taped

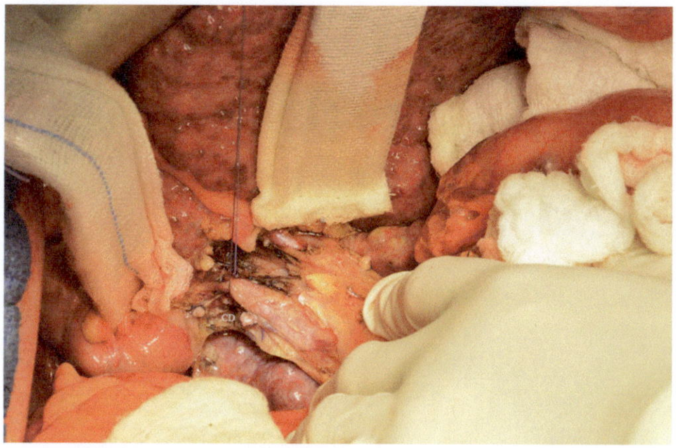

Fig. 3.8 Ligation of the common bile duct above the level of the cystic duct (CD)

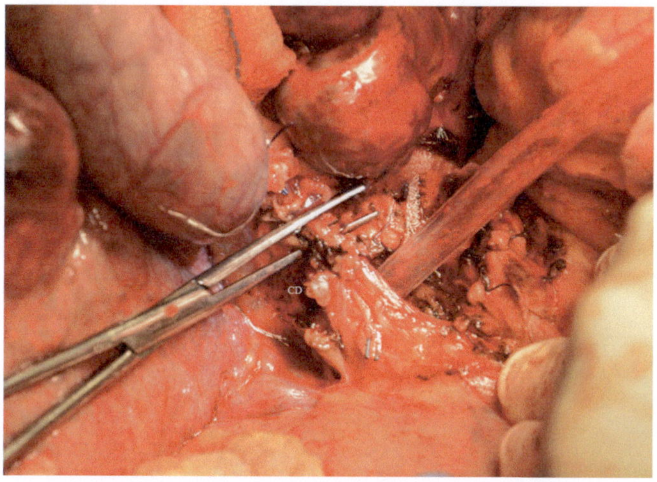

Fig. 3.9 Division of the common bile duct (CD, cystic duct)

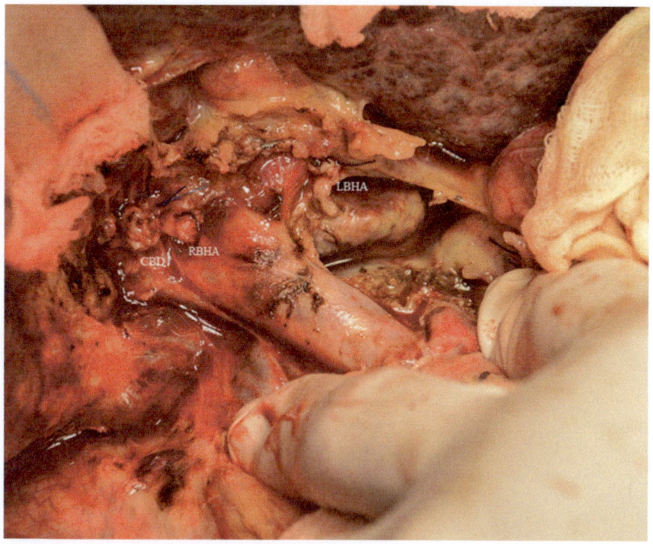

Fig. 3.10 After division of the hepatic artery and common bile duct, the portal vein is exposed (RBHA, right branch of the hepatic artery; LBHA, left branch of the hepatic artery; CBD, common bile duct)

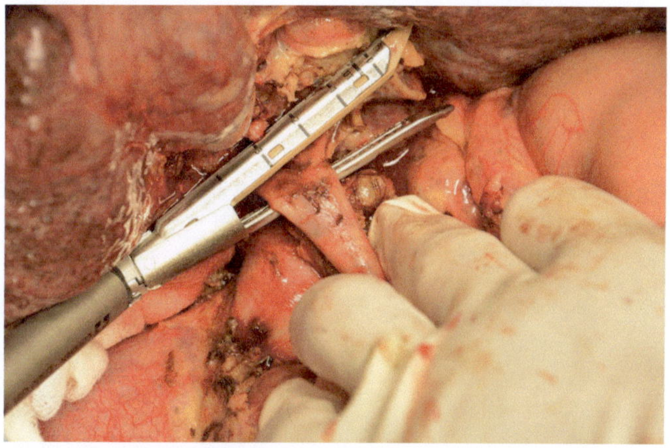

Fig. 3.11 The portal vein is divided using a vascular stapler

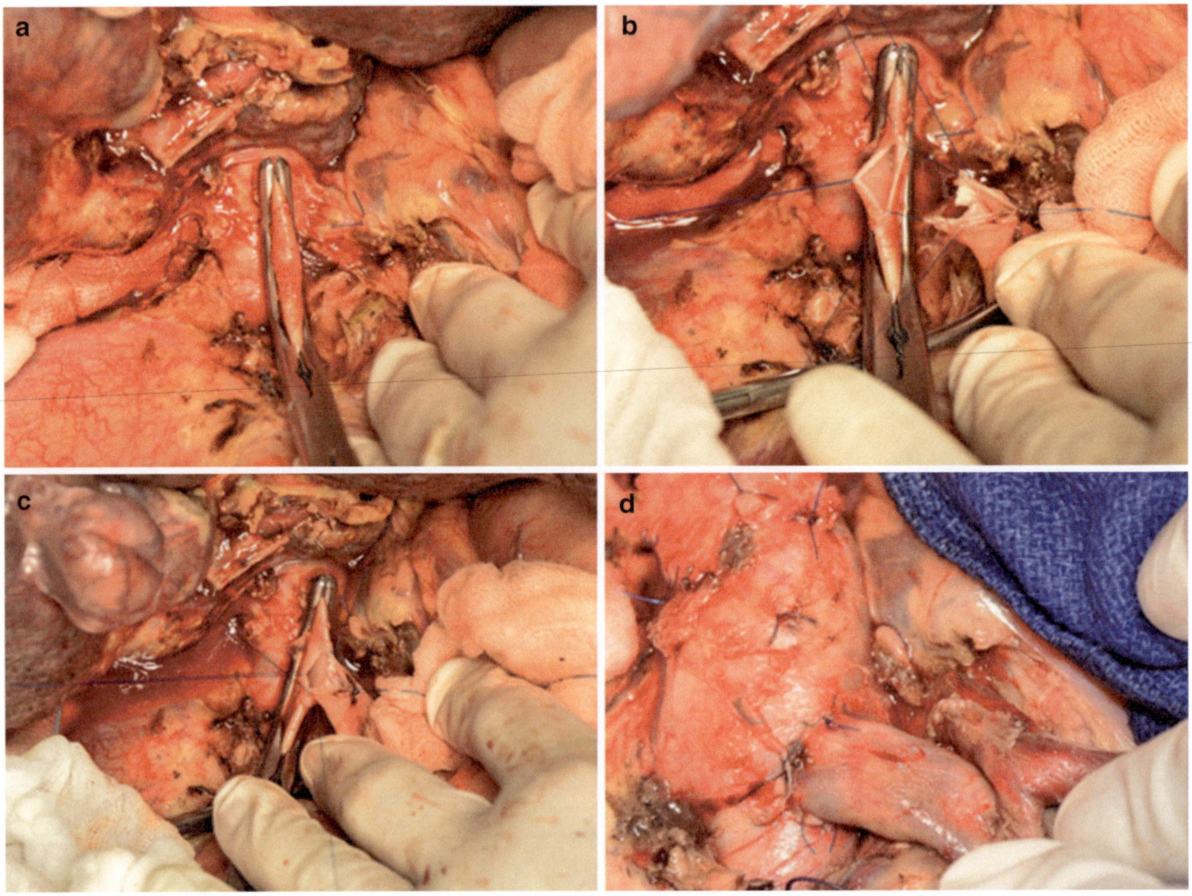

Fig. 3.12 Performing a temporary portocaval anastomosis. (**a**) The inferior vena cava is clamped laterally. (**b**) The inferior vena cava is opened. (**c**) The portal vein is anastomosed to the inferior vena cava. (**d**) Portocaval anastomosis after unclamping

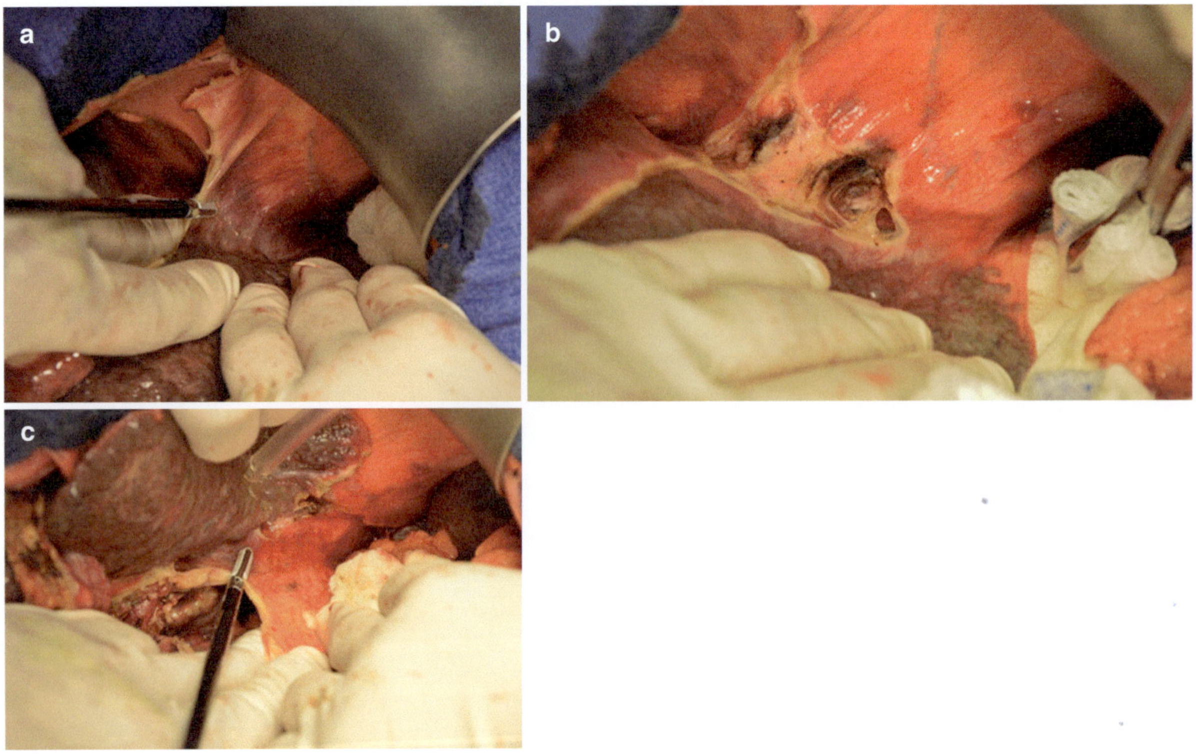

Fig. 3.13 Mobilization of the left liver. (**a**) Section of the falciform ligament. (**b**) Section of the left triangular ligament. (**c**) Section of the pars flaccida

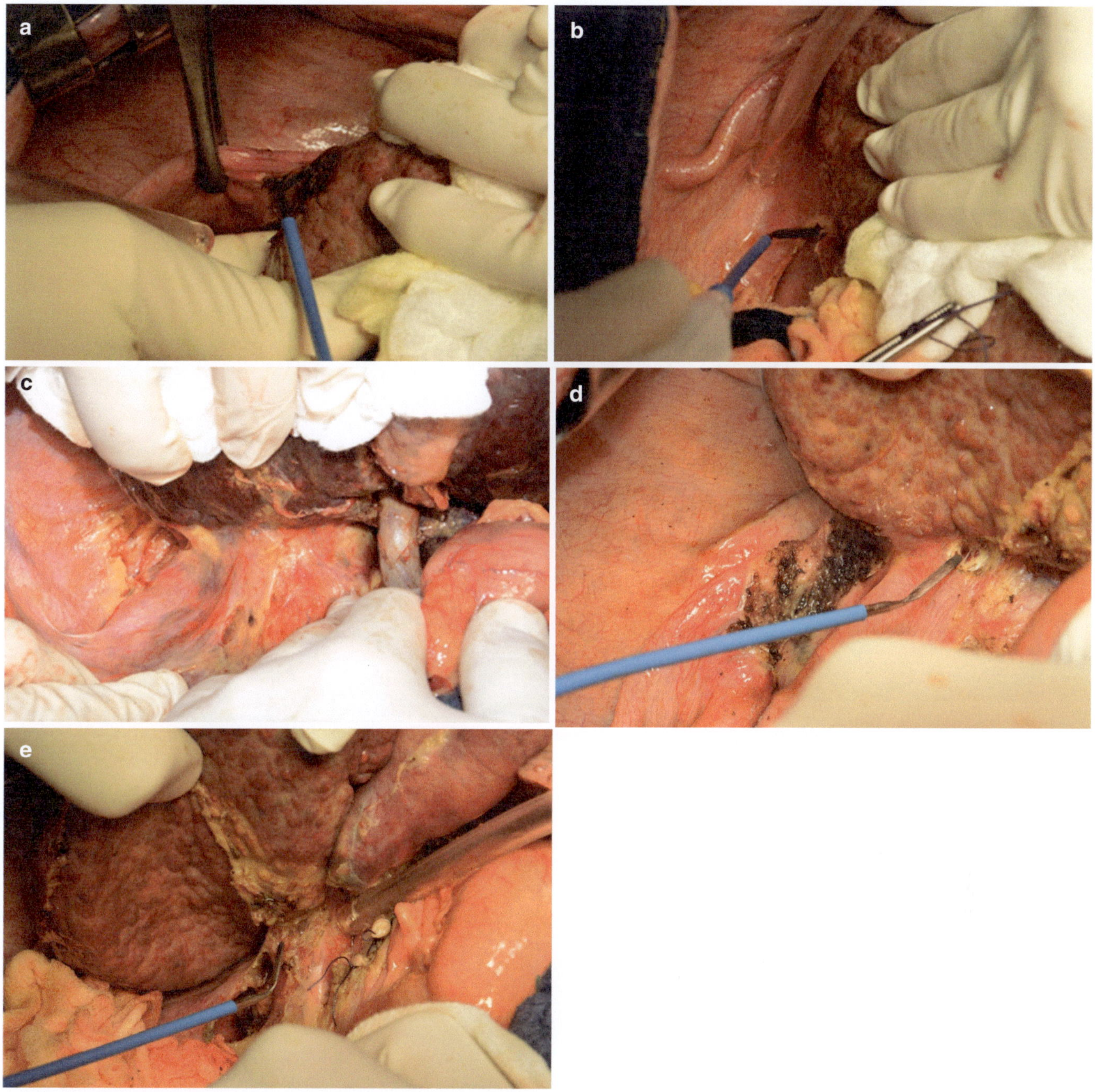

Fig. 3.14 Mobilization of the right liver. (**a**, **b**) Section of the right triangular ligament. (**c**–**e**) Exposition of the dorsal aspect of the right liver

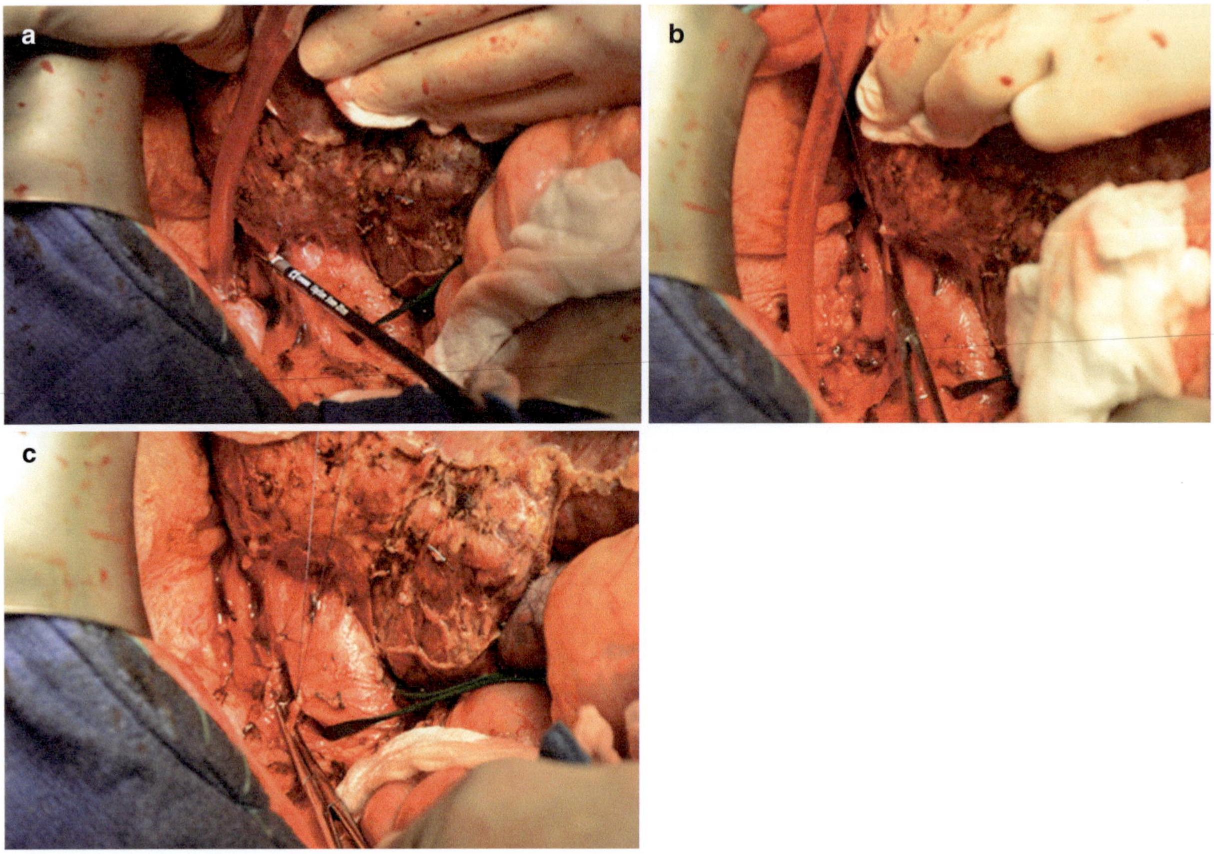

Fig. 3.15 The retrohepatic short veins are isolated, divided, and ligated caudo-cranially up to the root of the right hepatic vein (**a**–**c**)

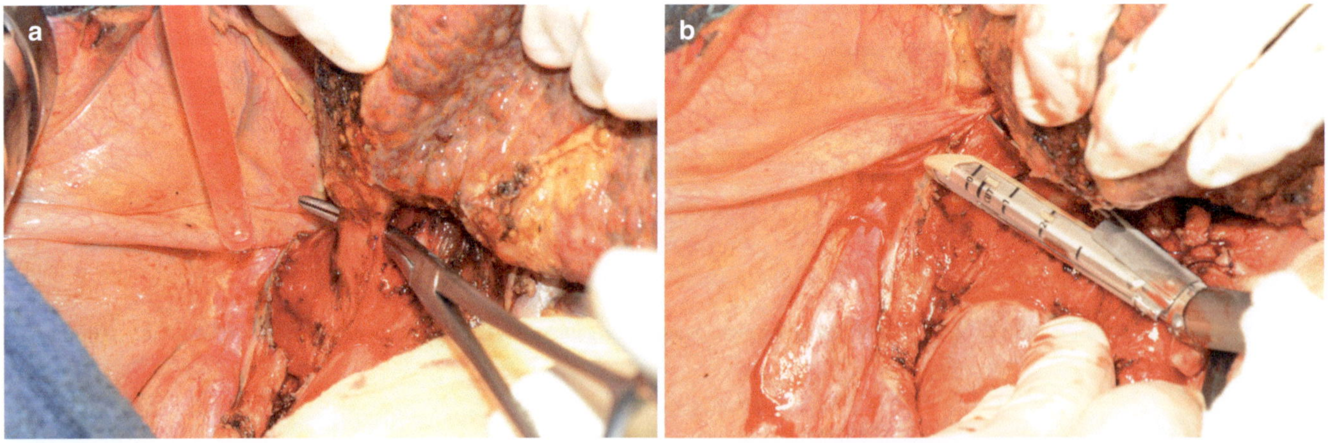

Fig. 3.16 Division of the hepatocaval ligament. (**a**) The hepatocaval ligament is isolated. (**b**) The hepatocaval ligament is divided using a vascular stapler

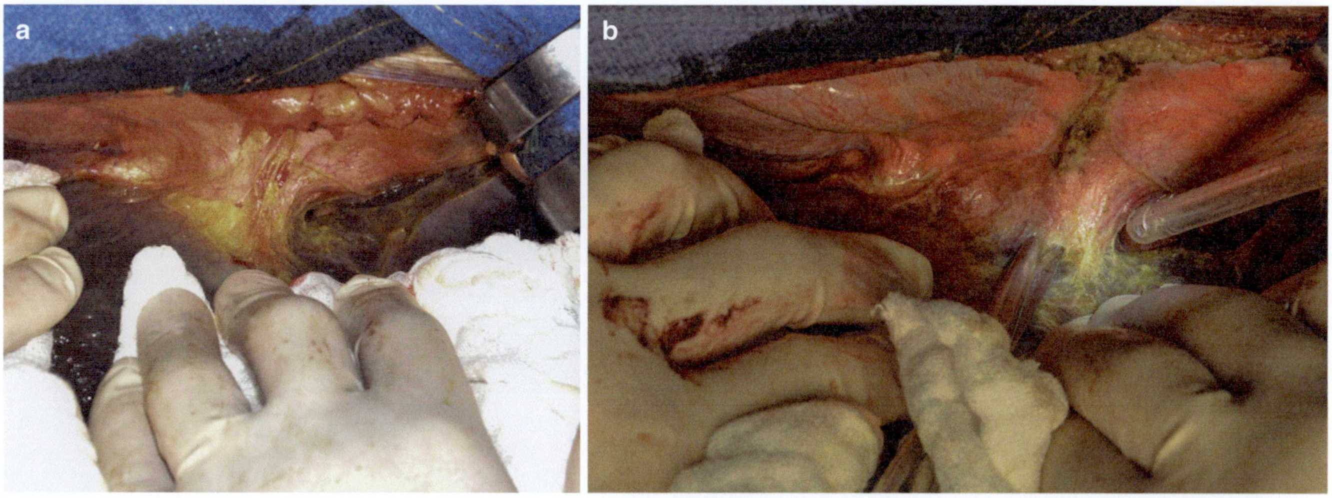

Fig. 3.17 Dissection of the hepatocaval confluence to expose the entry site of the hepatic veins into the suprahepatic inferior vena cava (**a**, **b**)

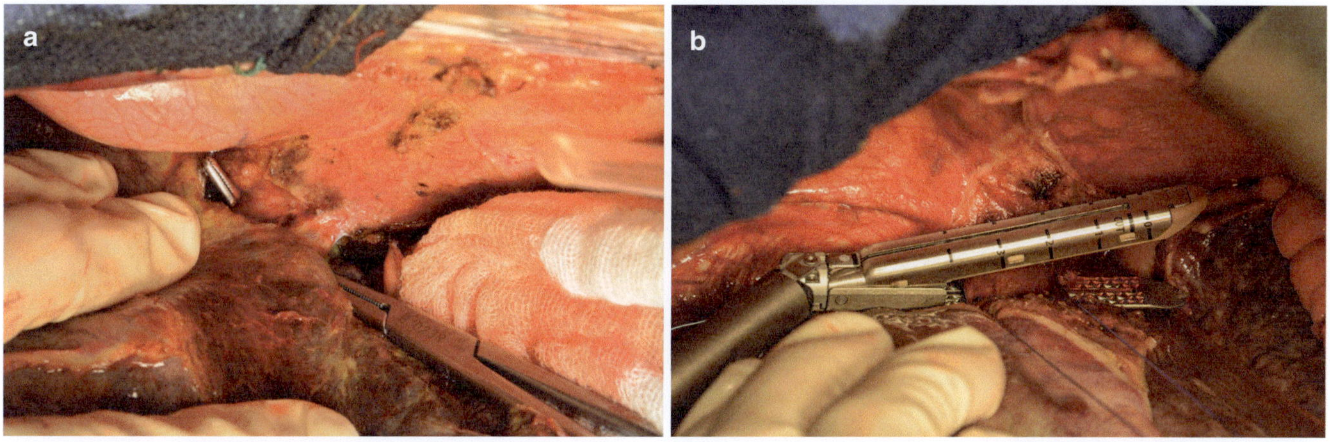

Fig. 3.18 The common trunk of the middle and left hepatic veins is controlled (**a**) and divided using a vascular stapler (**b**)

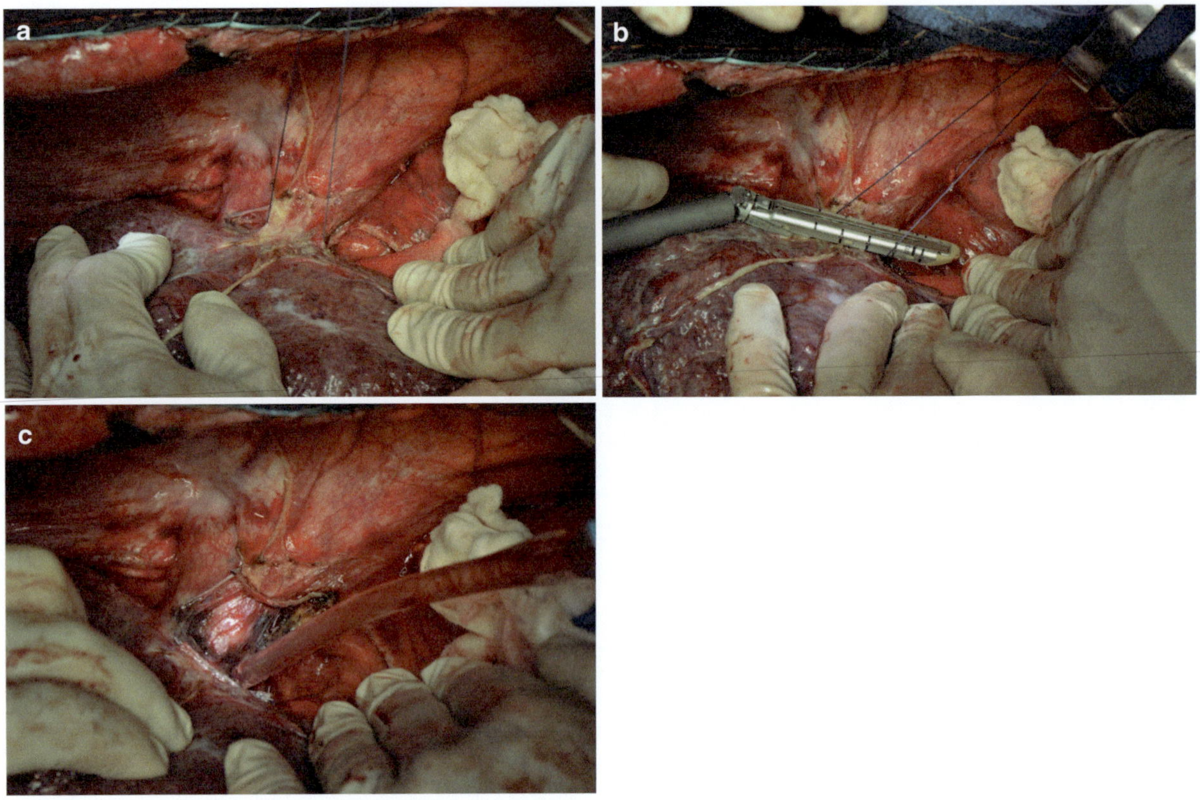

Fig. 3.19 The common trunk of the middle and left hepatic veins. (**a**) The common trunk of the middle and left hepatic veins is isolated (**a**) and divided using a vascular stapler (**b**, **c**)

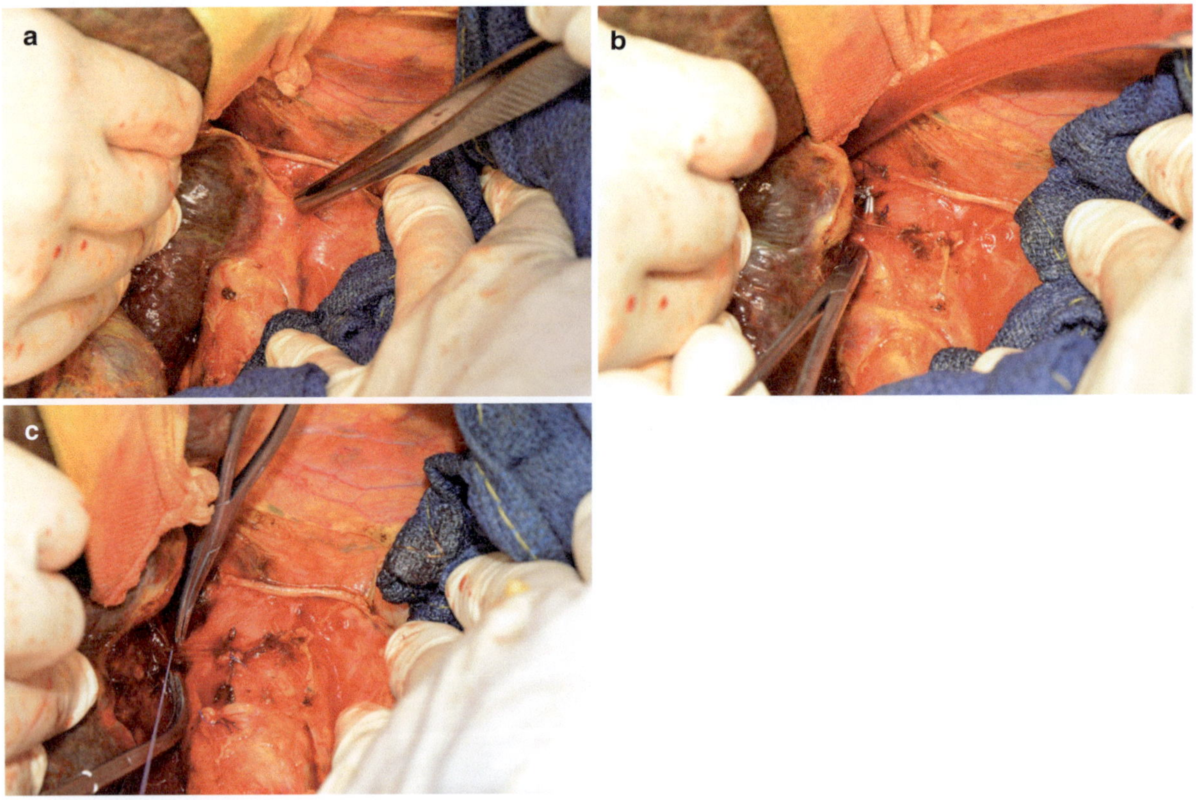

Fig. 3.20 Mobilization of the caudate lobe. The left-side area of the hepatocaval ligament is exposed (**a**). After division of the left side of the hepatocaval ligament, a vein of segment I is dissected (**b**) and divided (**c**)

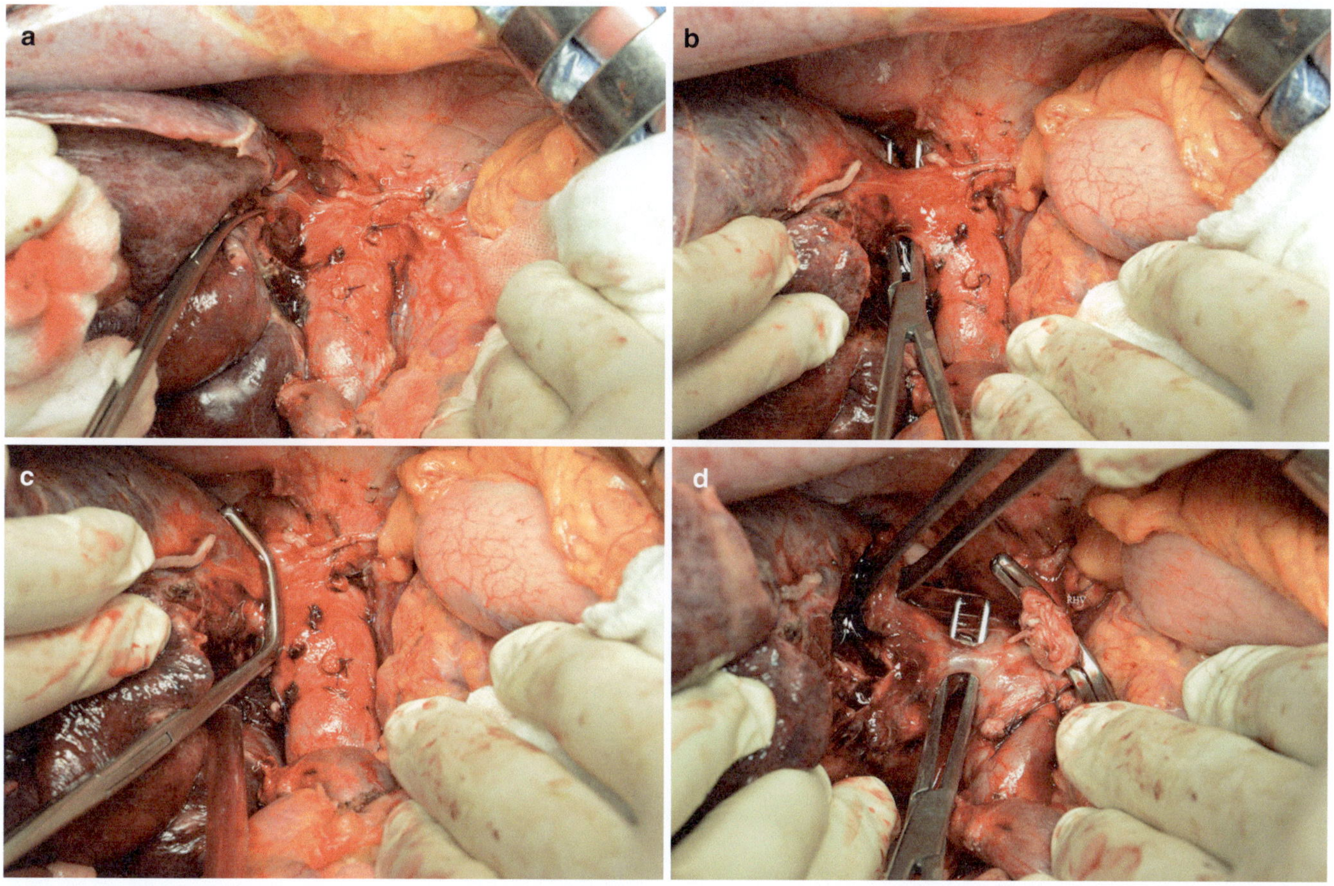

Fig. 3.21 Total hepatectomy from the left to the right. After division of the common trunk, the anterior and left parts of the inferior vena cava are totally exposed (**a**). The right hepatic vein is dissected (**b**) and divided (**c**). A retrohepatic vein of segment VII is dissected (**d**)

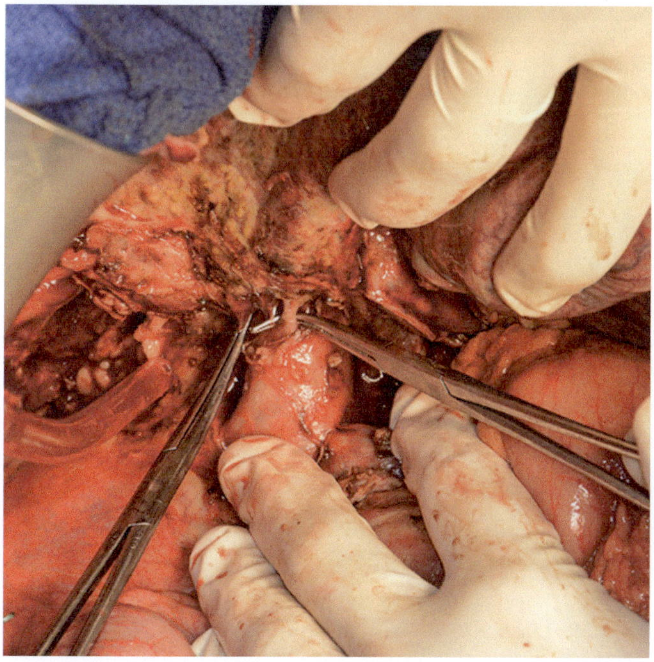

Fig. 3.22 Dissection of a retrohepatic vein before total hepatectomy

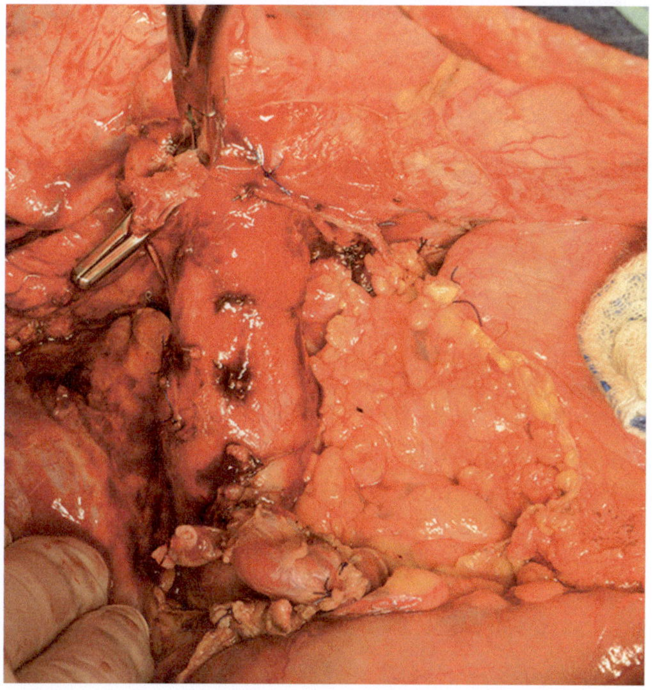

Fig. 3.23 The inferior vena cava is totally exposed after total hepatectomy

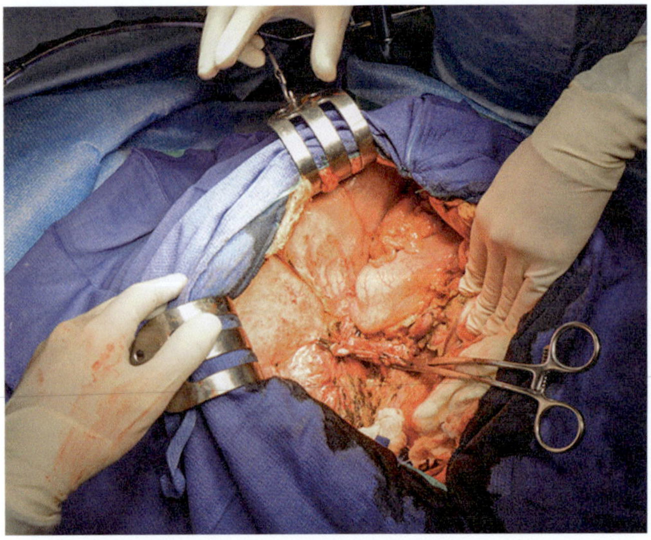

Fig. 3.24 Completion of the total hepatectomy stage

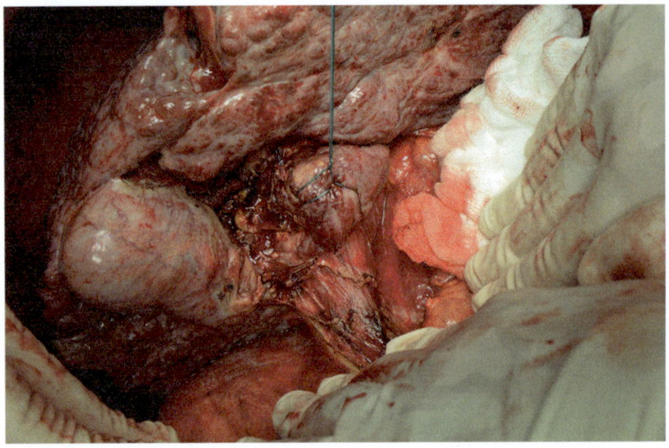

Fig. 3.25 Mobilization of the caudate lobe from the inferior vena cava

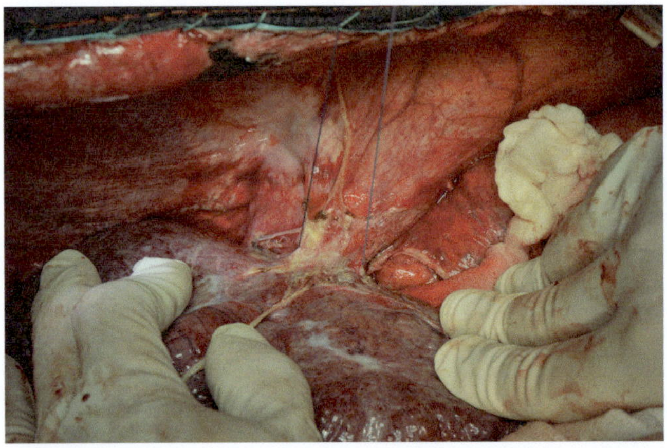

Fig. 3.26 Control of the common trunk of the middle and left hepatic veins

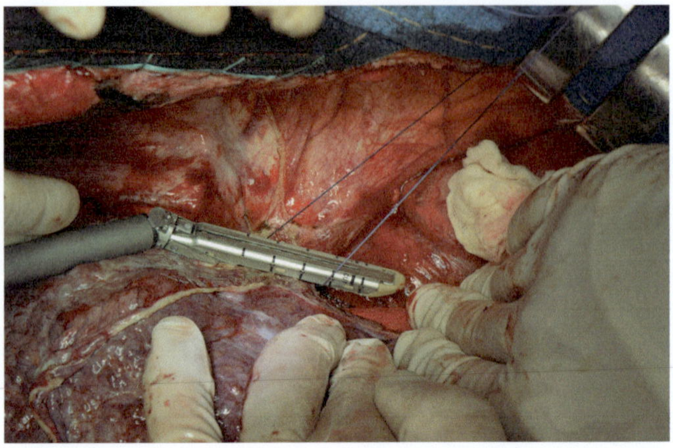

Fig. 3.27 Section of the common trunk of the middle and left hepatic veins using a vascular stapler

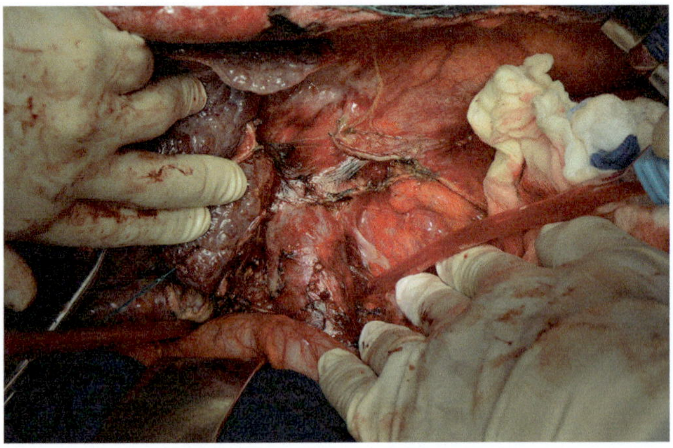

Fig. 3.28 Total mobilization of the caudate lobe and section of the common trunk of the middle and left hepatic veins

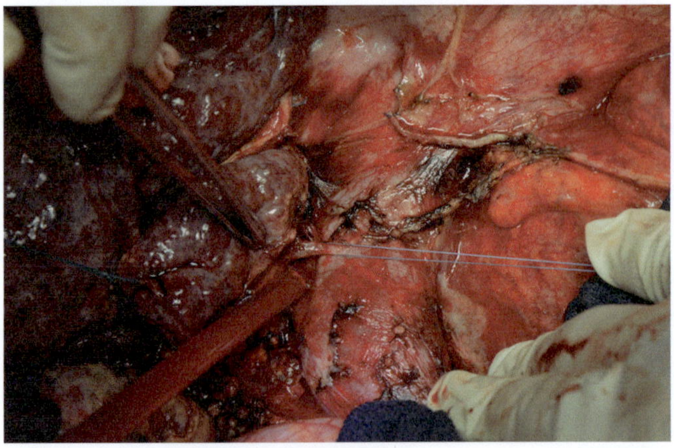

Fig. 3.29 Ligation of a vein from the caudate lobe

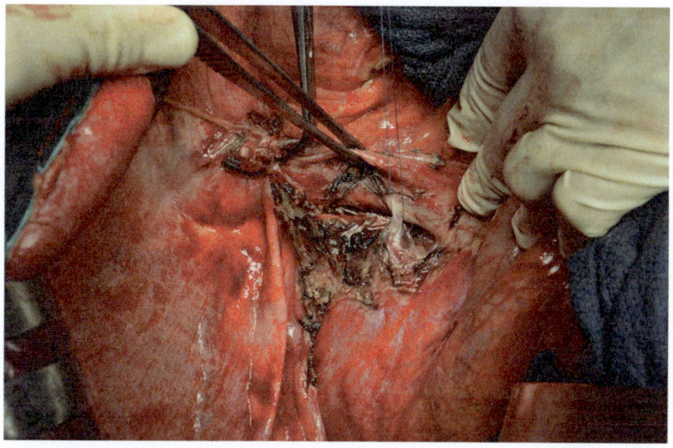

Fig. 3.30 After total hepatectomy, mobilization of the inferior vena cava with control of the right adrenal vein

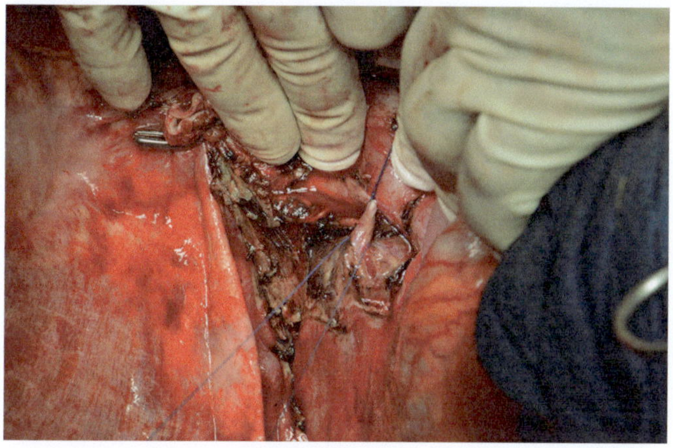

Fig. 3.31 After total hepatectomy, mobilization of the inferior vena cava with ligation of the right adrenal vein

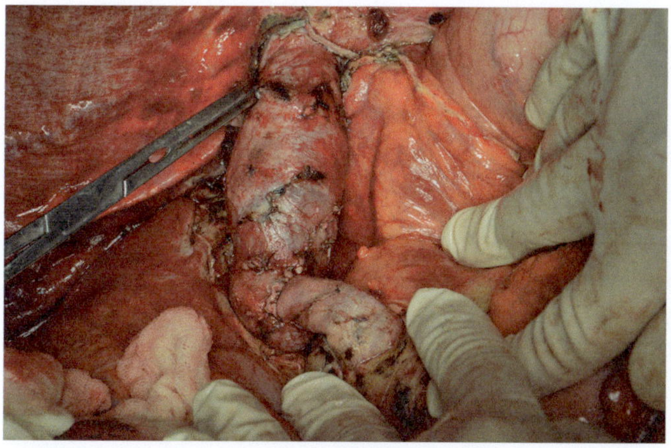

Fig. 3.32 Completion of the total hepatectomy stage in the presence of a portocaval shunt and clamping of the right hepatic vein

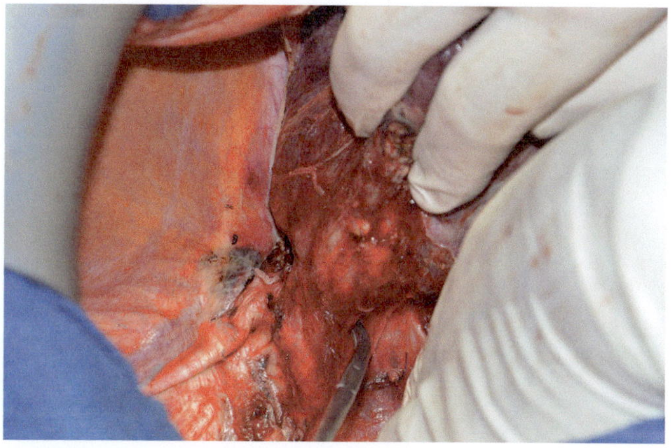

Fig. 3.33 Total hepatectomy from the right to the left: control of the hepatocaval ligament

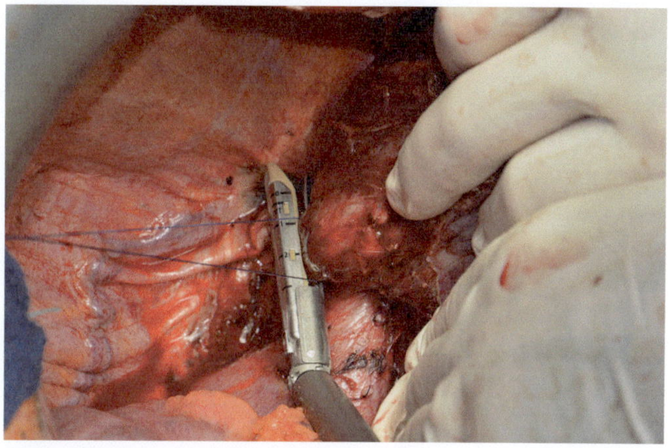

Fig. 3.34 Total hepatectomy from the right to the left: division of the hepatocaval ligament

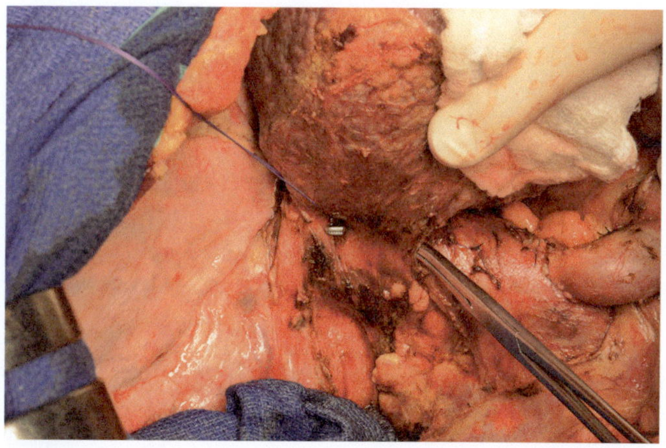

Fig. 3.35 Total hepatectomy from the right to the left: control of the inferior right hepatic vein

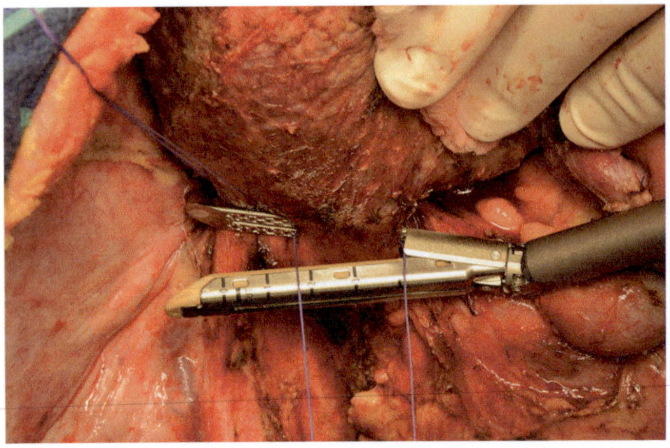

Fig. 3.36 Total hepatectomy from the right to the left: division of the inferior right hepatic vein

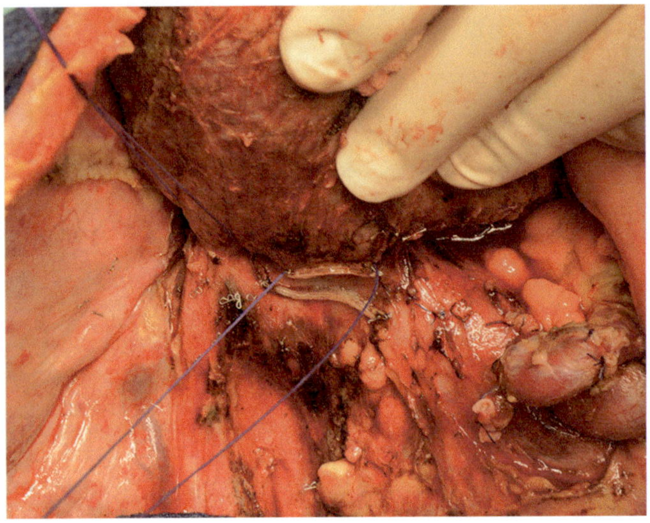

Fig. 3.37 Total hepatectomy from the right to the left: after division of the inferior right hepatic vein

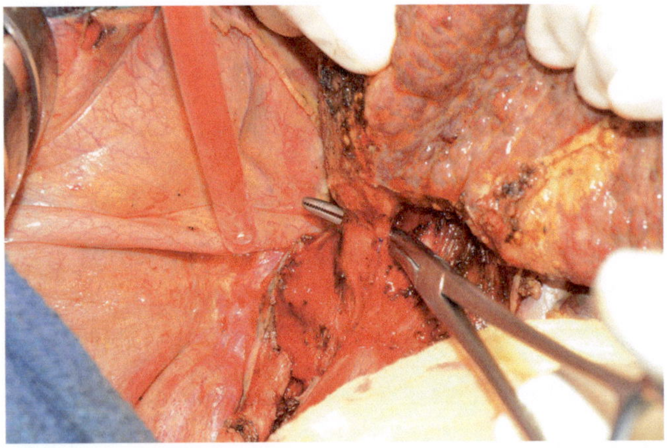

Fig. 3.38 Total hepatectomy from the right to the left: control of the right hepatic vein

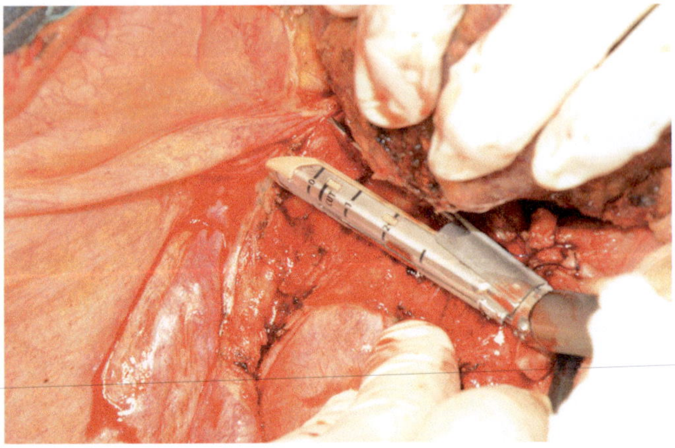

Fig. 3.39 Total hepatectomy from the right to the left: division of the right hepatic vein

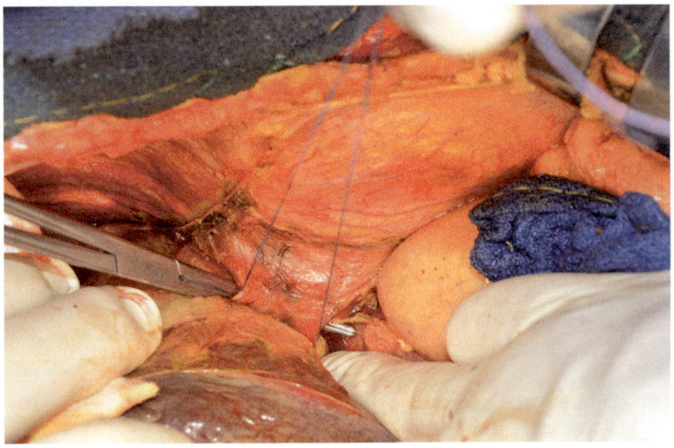

Fig. 3.40 Total hepatectomy from the right to the left: control of the common trunk

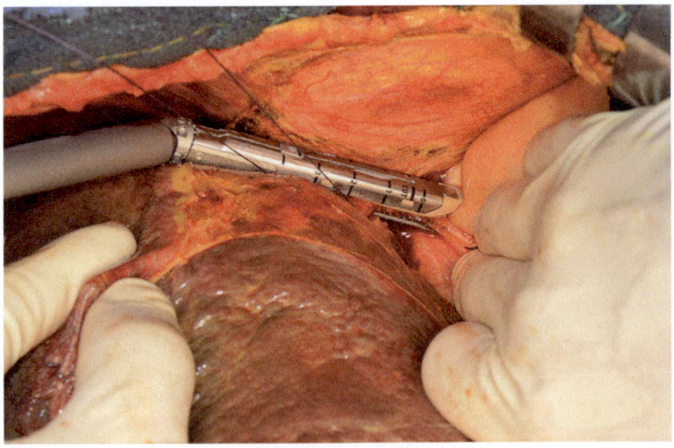

Fig. 3.41 Total hepatectomy from the right to the left: division of the common trunk

References

1. Calne RY, Williams R. Liver transplantation in man. I. Observations on technique and organization in five cases. Br Med J. 1968;4(5630):535–40.
2. Belghiti J. Preservation of portacaval flow in liver transplantation: a technical progress originating from hepatic surgery. Ann Chir. 1994:48(11):989–90. PMID: 7733606.
3. Belghiti J, Noun R, Sauvanet A. Temporary portocaval anastomosis with preservation of caval flow during orthotopic liver transplantation. Am J Surg. 1995:169(2):277–9. https://doi.org/10.1016/S0002-9610(99)80151-2. PMID: 7840394
4. Belghiti J, Noun R, Sauvanet A, Durand F, Aschehoug J, Erlinger S, Benhamou JP, Bernuau J. Transplantation for fulminant and subfulminant hepatic failure with preservation of portal and caval flow. Br J Surg. 1995:82(7):986–9. https://doi.org/10.1002/bjs.1800820741. PMID: 7648127.
5. Belghiti J, Ettorre GM, Durand F, Sommacale D, Sauvanet A, Jerius JT, Farges O. Feasibility and limits of caval-flow preservation during liver transplantation. Liver Transpl. 2001:7(11):983–7. https://doi.org/10.1053/jlts.2001.28242. PMID: 11699035.
6. Dondéro F, Liddo G, Andraus W, Sommacale D, Sauvanet A, Belghiti J. Left-to-right approach facilitates total hepatectomy with caval flow preservation. Liver Transpl. 2008:14(9):1380–2. https://doi.org/10.1002/lt.21503. PMID: 18756489.
7. Tzakis A, Todo S, Starzl TE. Orthotopic liver transplantation with preservation of the inferior vena cava. Ann Surg. 1989;210(5):649–52. https://doi.org/10.1097/00000658-198911000-00013.

Standard Vascular and Biliary Reconstructions

4

During implantation of the graft, the continuity of each anastomosis is restored. In case of orthotopic liver transplantation with preservation of the caval flow, several methods of graft-to-inferior vena cava implantation are possible (side-to-side, end-to-side, two- or three-vein piggyback anastomosis). Standard portal reconstruction was defined by graft portal vein to native portal vein anastomosis. Standard arterial reconstruction was defined by graft hepatic artery to native hepatic artery anastomosis [1]. Standard biliary reconstruction was defined by biliary-biliary anastomosis (Figs. 4.1, 4.2, 4.3, 4.4, 4.5, 4.6, 4.7, 4.8, 4.9, 4.10, 4.11, 4.12, 4.13, 4.14, 4.15, 4.16, 4.17, 4.18, 4.19, 4.20, 4.21, 4.22, 4.23, 4.24, and 4.25).

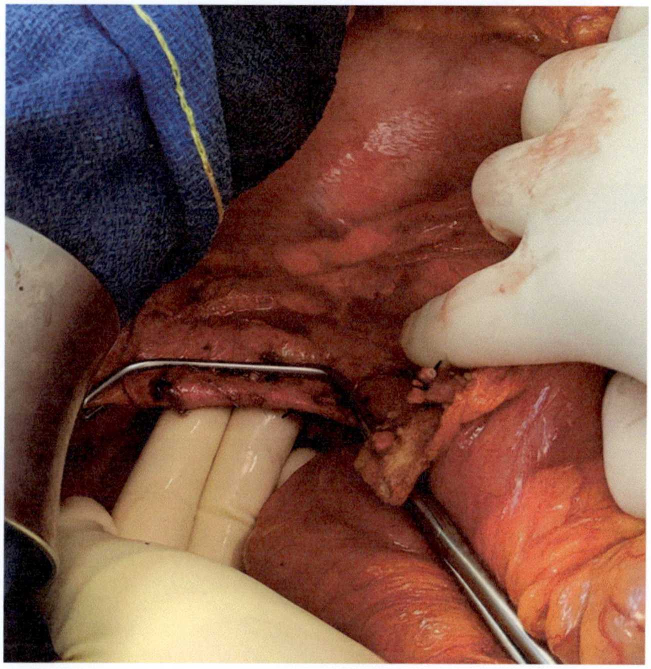

Fig. 4.1 Lateral clamping of the inferior vena cava

C. Lim et al., *Atlas of Liver Transplantation*, https://doi.org/10.1007/978-3-031-85264-0_4

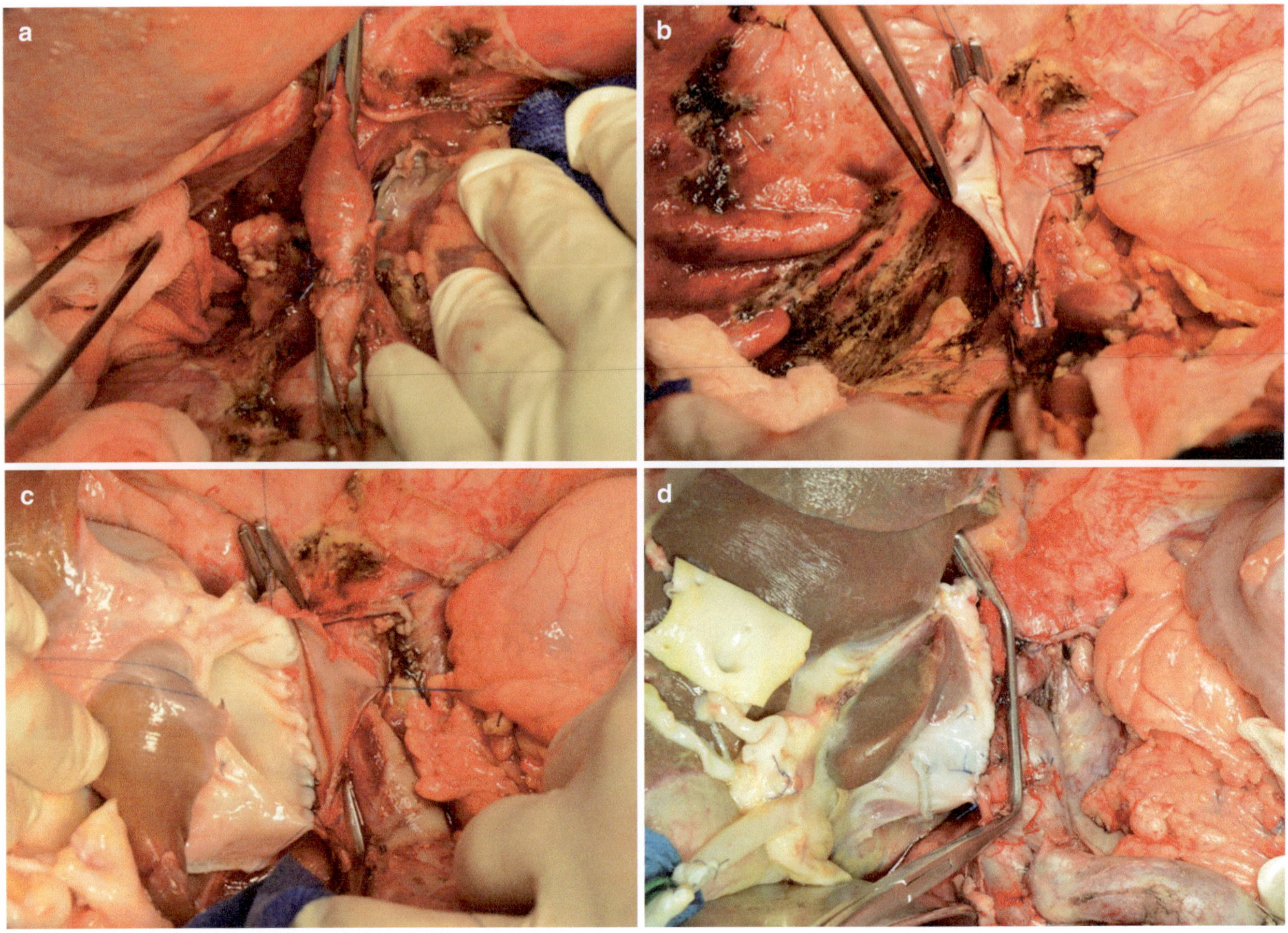

Fig. 4.2 Side-to-side caval anastomosis. (**a**) Lateral clamping of the native inferior vena cava. (**b**) Incision of the anterior wall of the native inferior vena cava. (**c**) Anastomose of the back caval wall with a running Prolene 4.0 suture. (**d**) Completion of the side-to-side anastomosis before unclamping

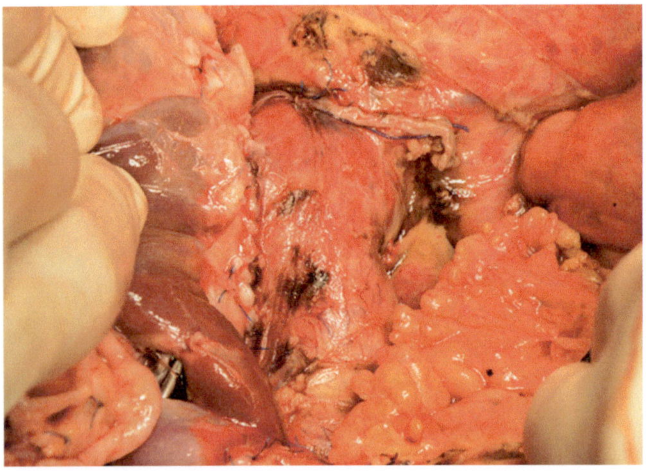

Fig. 4.3 Side-to-side caval anastomosis after unclamping

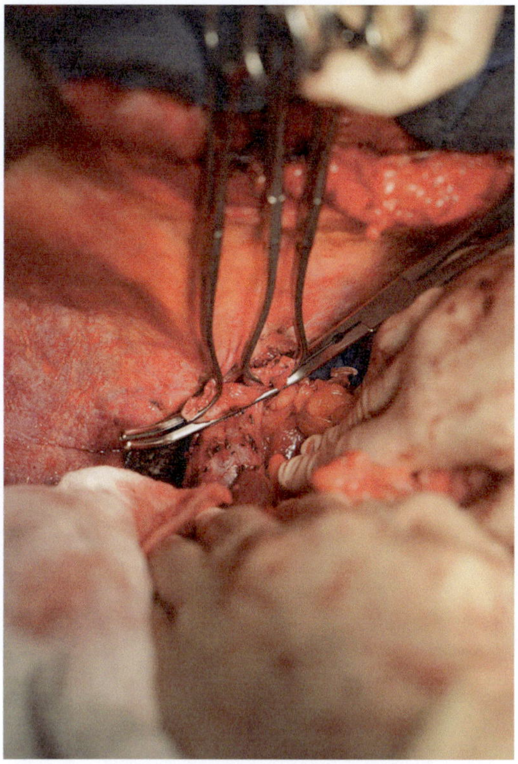

Fig. 4.4 The three-vein piggyback anastomosis: the three vascular clamps are held in line and retracted ventrally. A large Satinsky clamp is placed at the junction of the hepatic veins and the vena cava

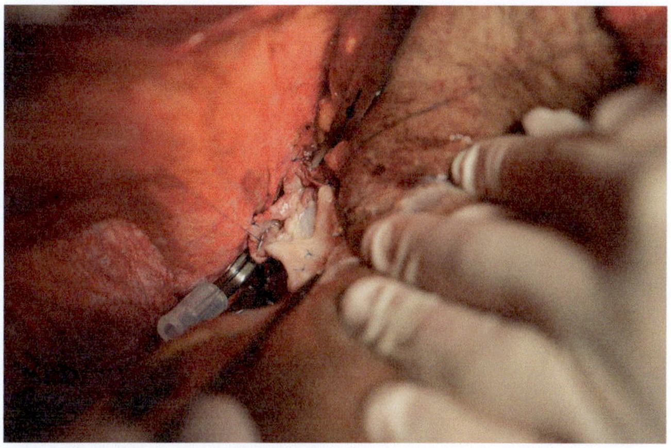

Fig. 4.5 The three-vein piggyback anastomosis: anastomose the back caval wall with a running Prolene 4.0 suture

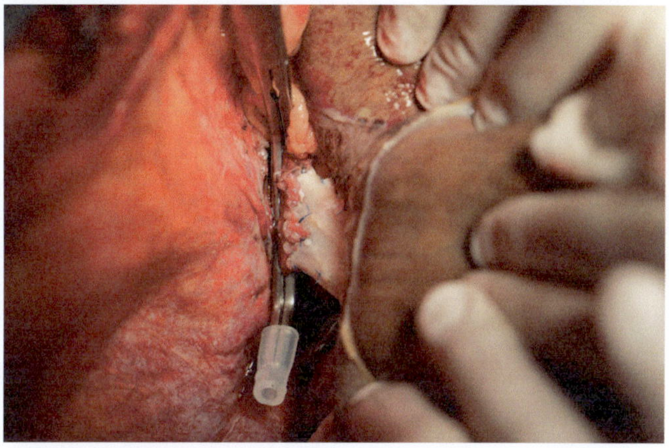

Fig. 4.6 The three-vein piggyback anastomosis: anastomose the front caval wall with another running Prolene 4.0 suture

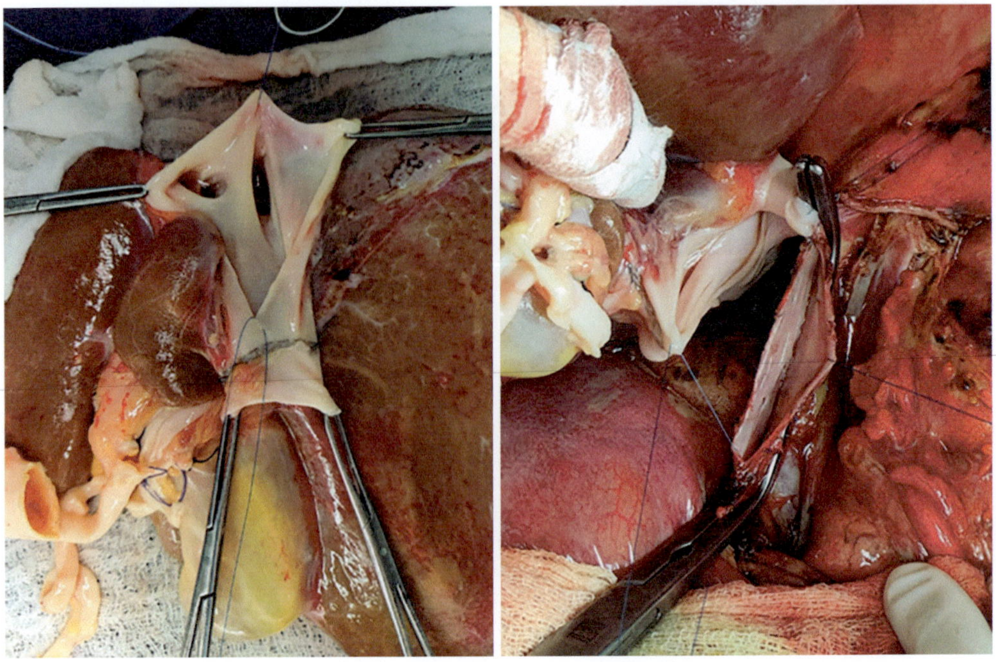

Fig. 4.7 End-to-side caval anastomosis

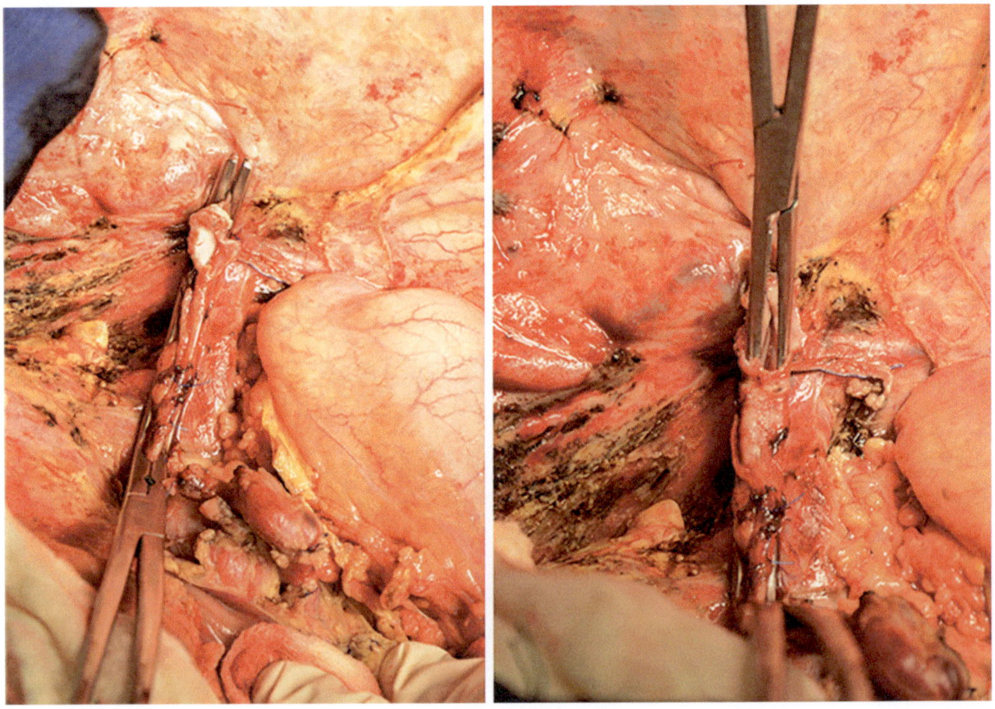

Fig. 4.8 Incision of the anterior wall of the native inferior vena cava including the right hepatic vein

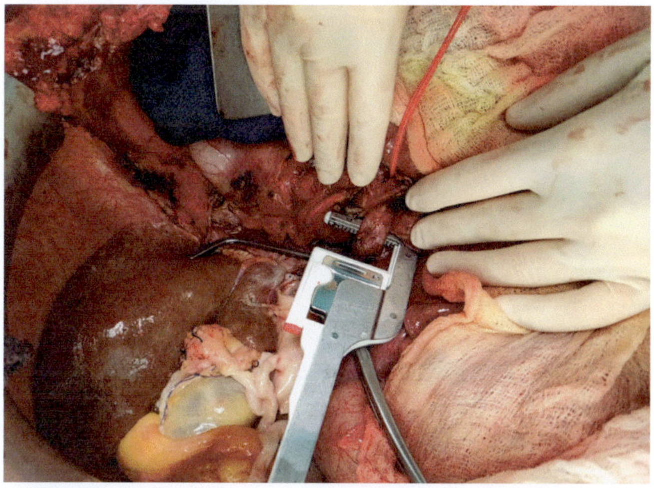

Fig. 4.9 Closure of the temporary end-to-side portocaval anastomosis before portal anastomosis using a vascular stapler

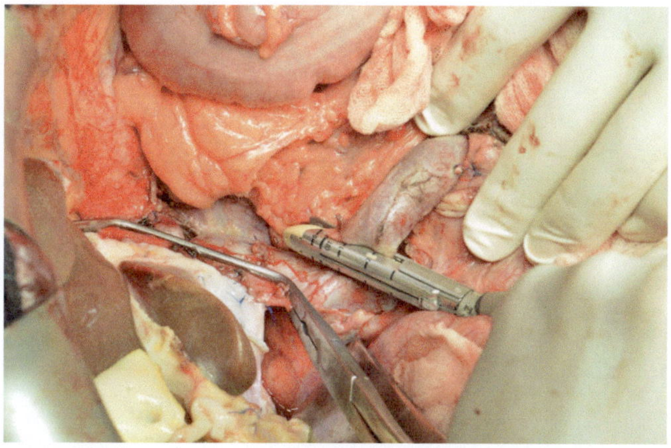

Fig. 4.10 Closure of the temporary end-to-side portocaval anastomosis before portal anastomosis using a vascular stapler

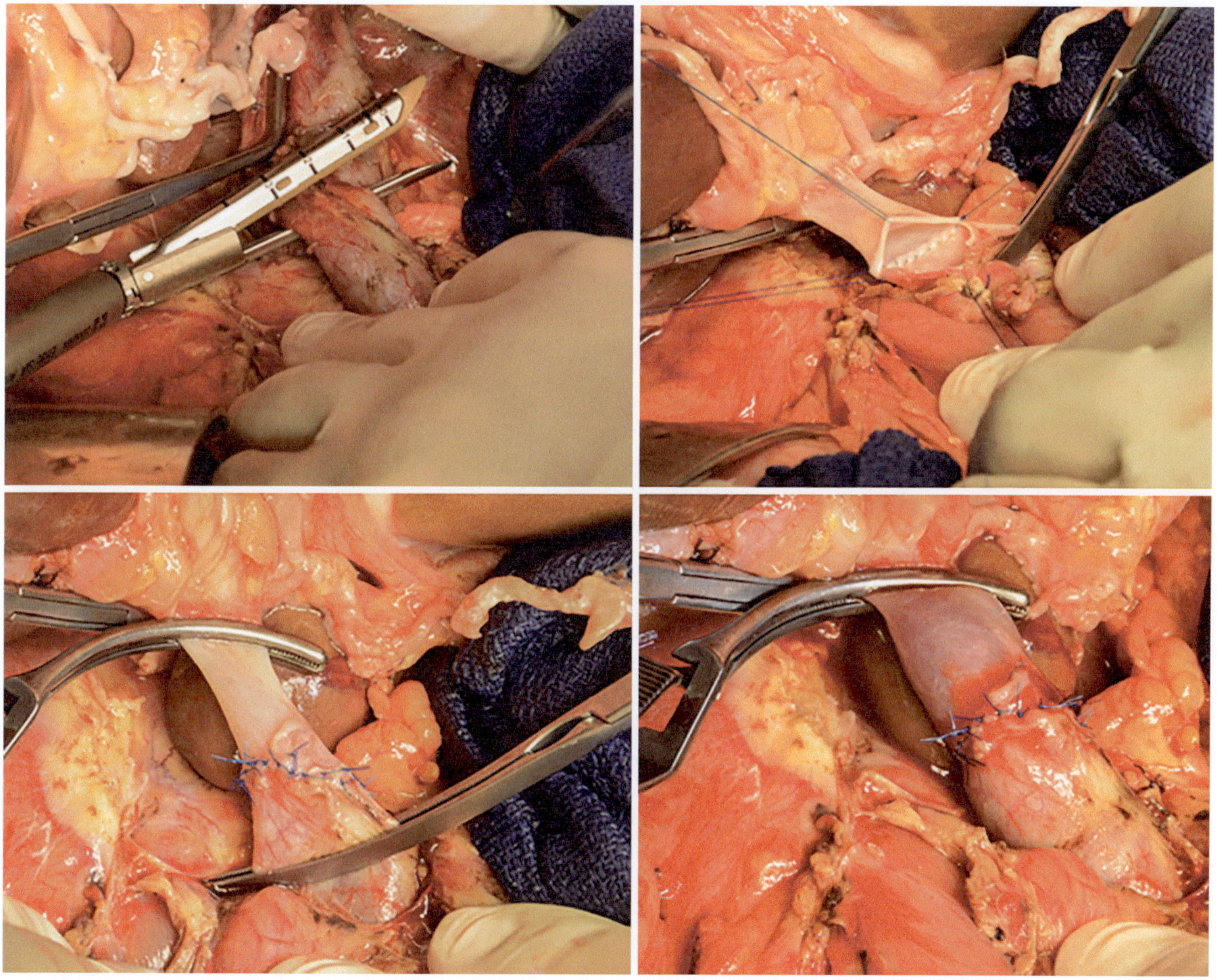

Fig. 4.11 Portoportal anastomosis: section of the temporary end-to-side portocaval anastomosis, completion of the portoportal anastomosis, and unclamping

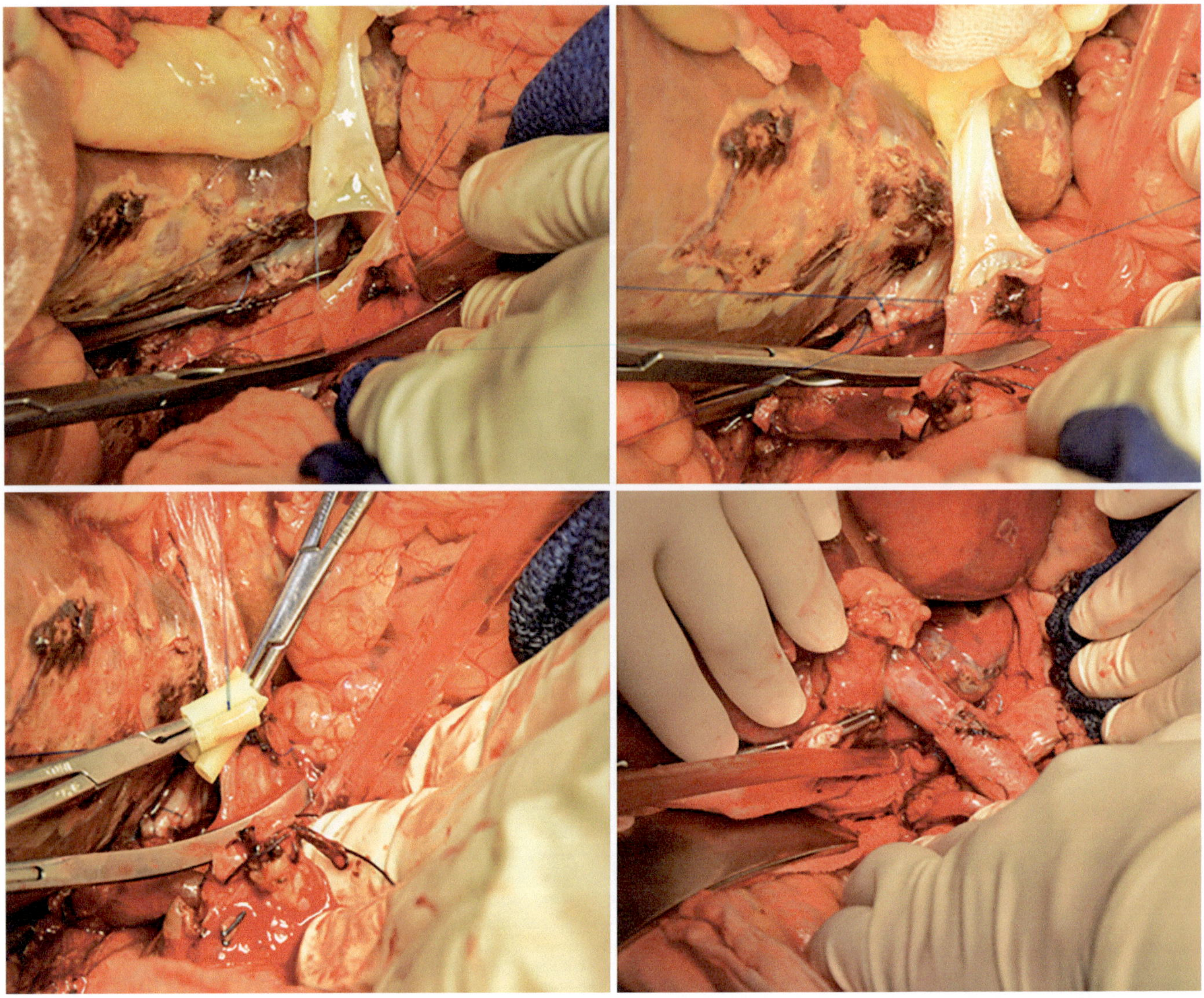

Fig. 4.12 Portoportal anastomosis with the growth factor

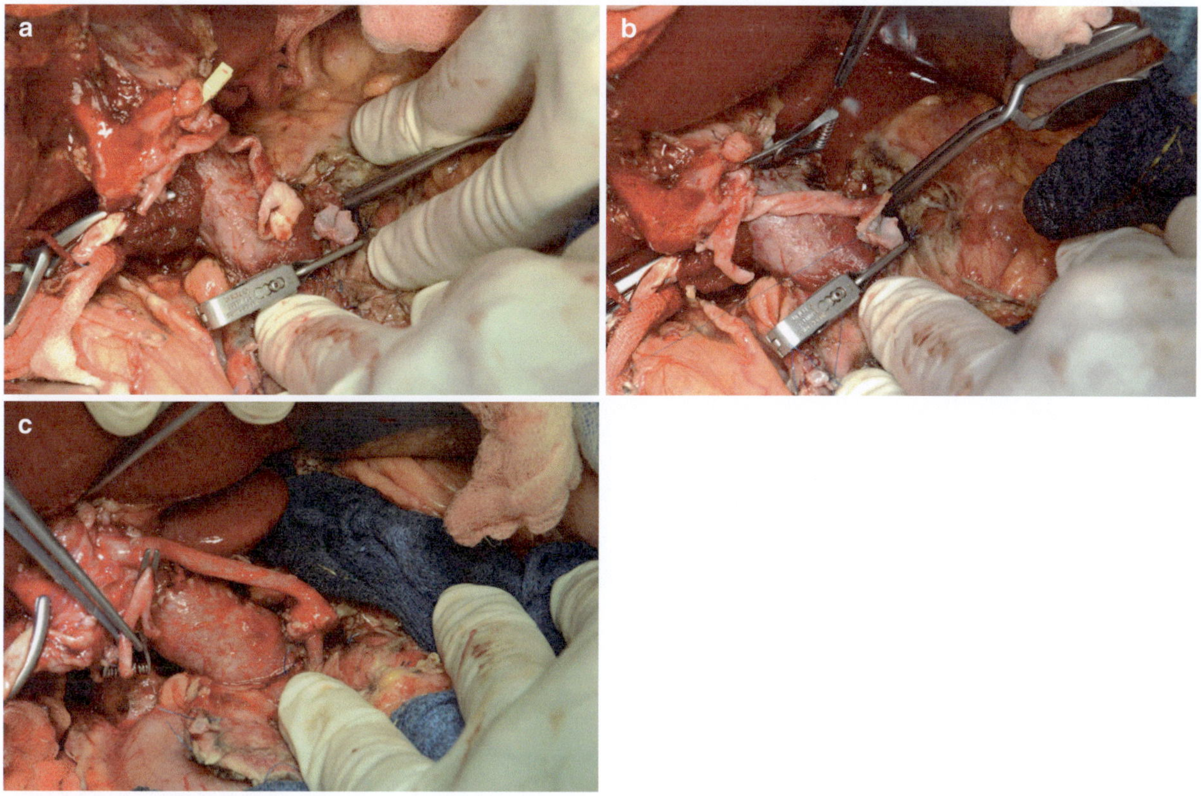

Fig. 4.13 Arterial anastomosis (**a**–**c**)

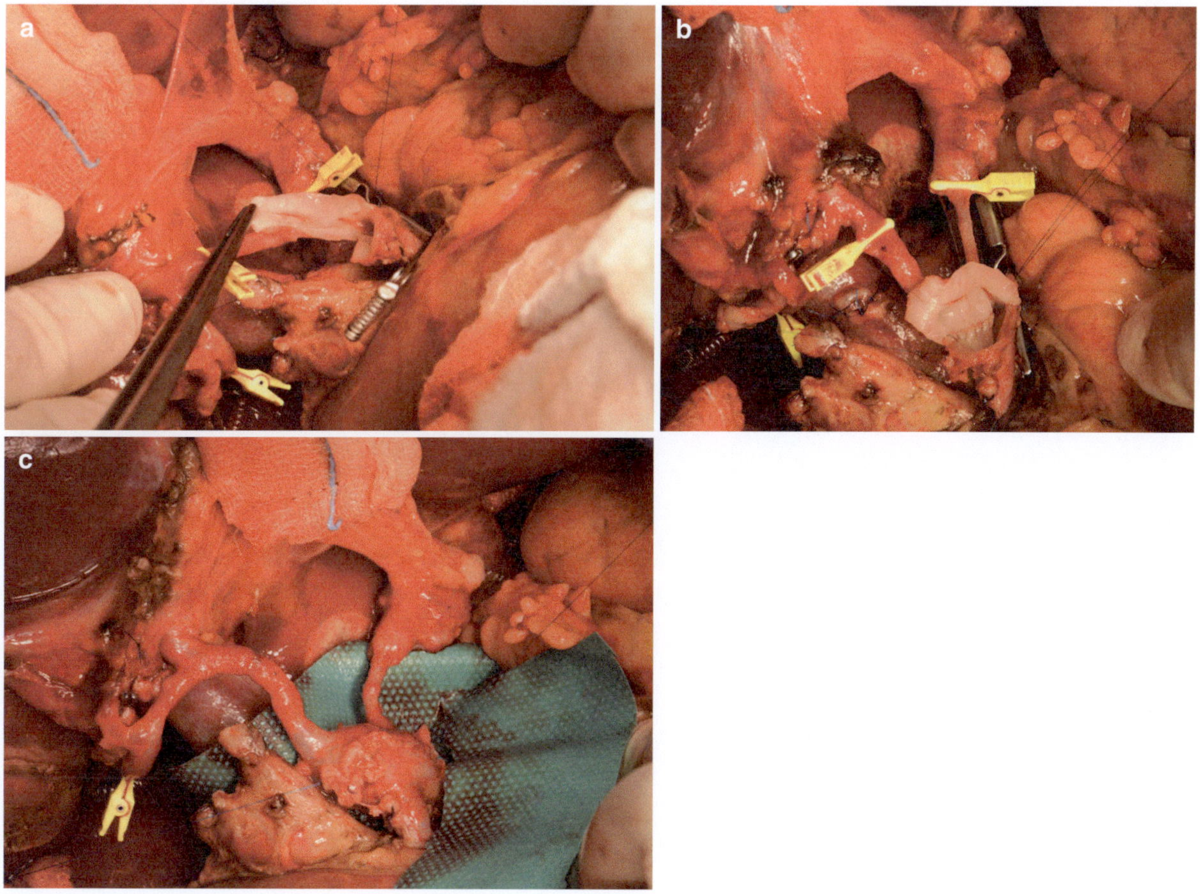

Fig. 4.14 Arterial anastomosis (**a**–**c**)

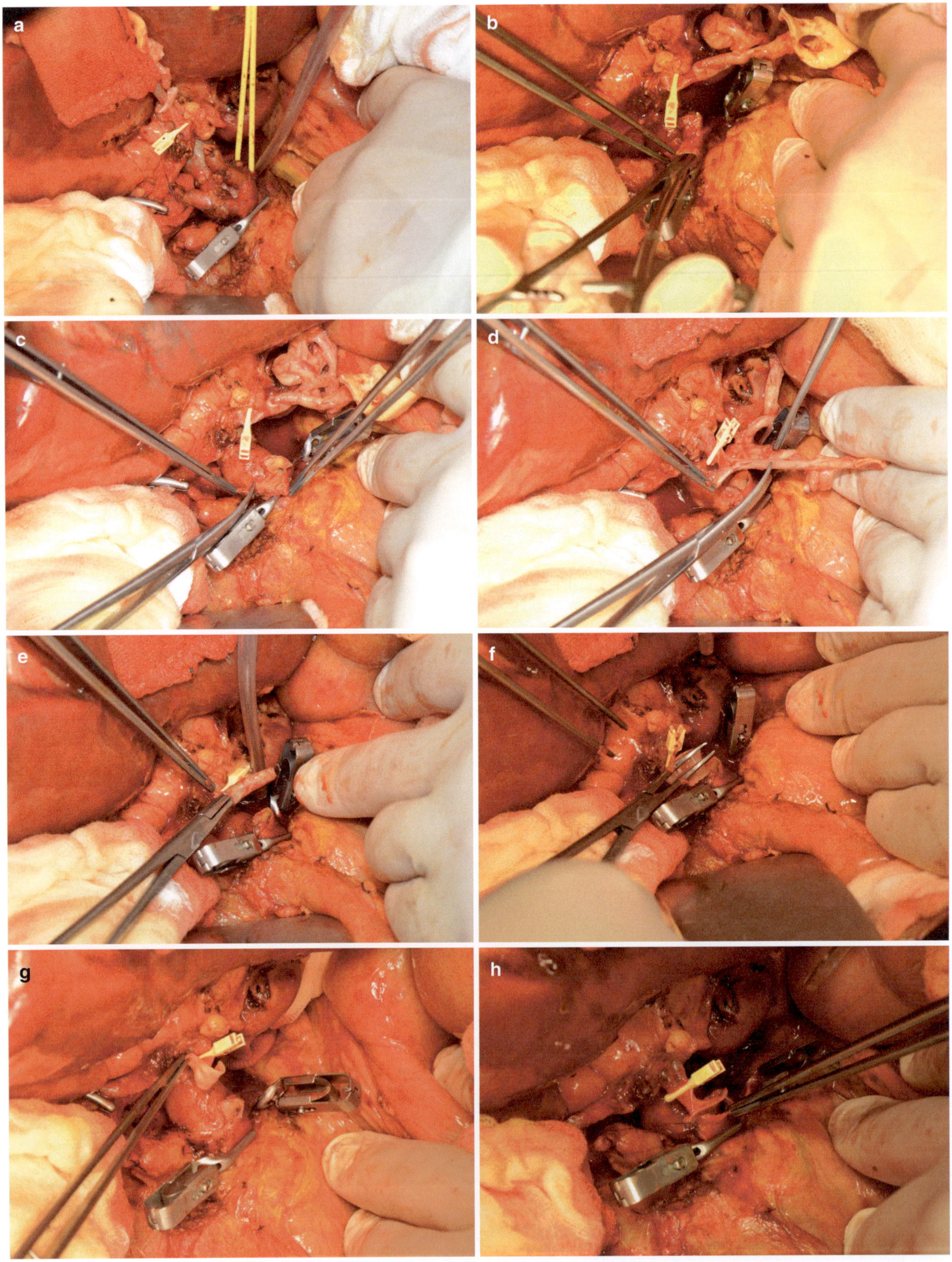

Fig. 4.15 Arterial anastomosis (**a–i**)

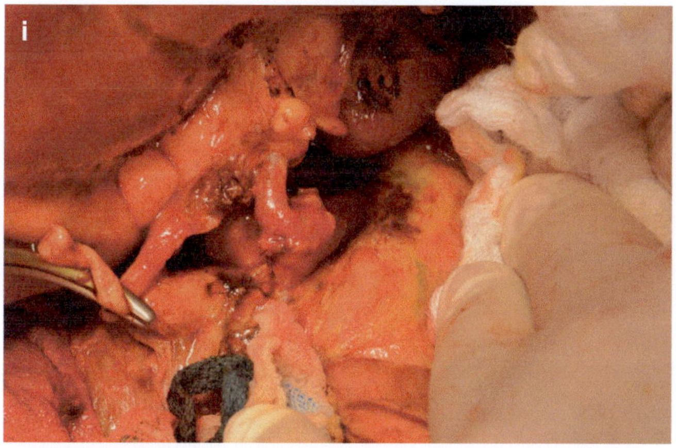

Fig. 4.15 (continued)

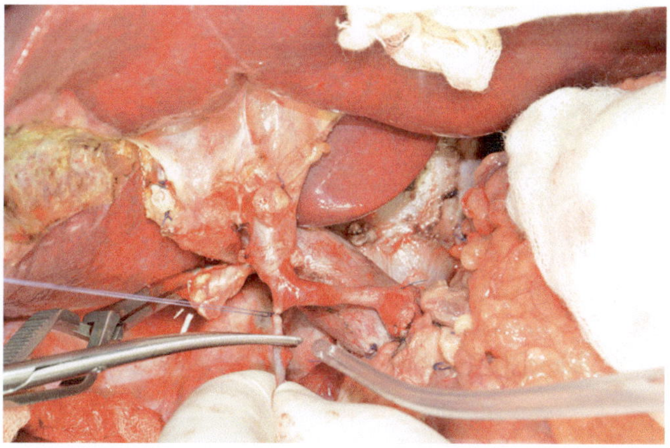

Fig. 4.16 Ligation of the graft gastroduodenal artery

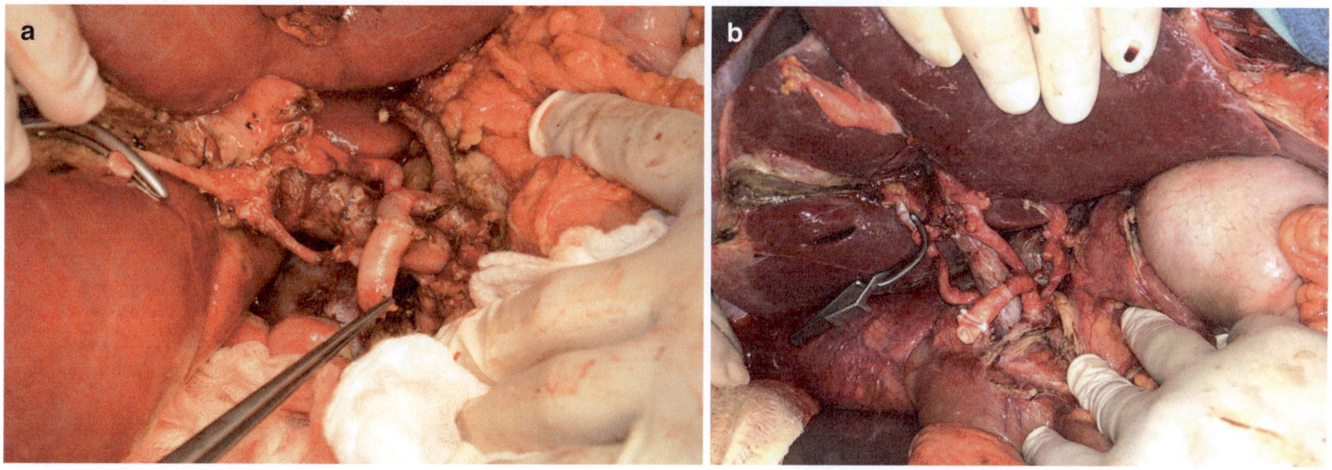

Fig. 4.17 Liver graft with two arteries: a replaced right hepatic artery arising from the superior mesenteric artery and a common hepatic artery (**a**, **b**)

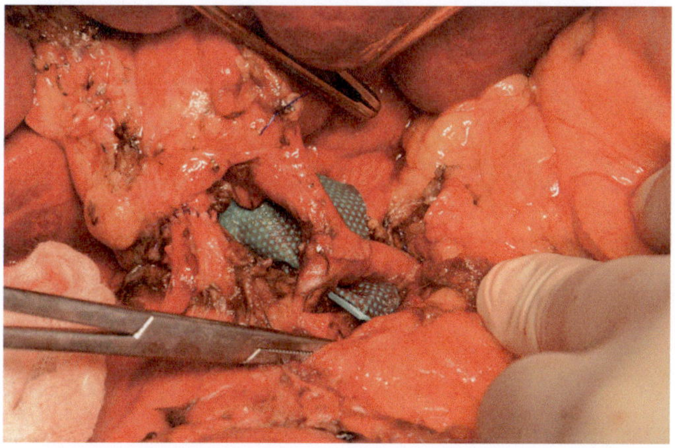

Fig. 4.18 Arterial anastomosis

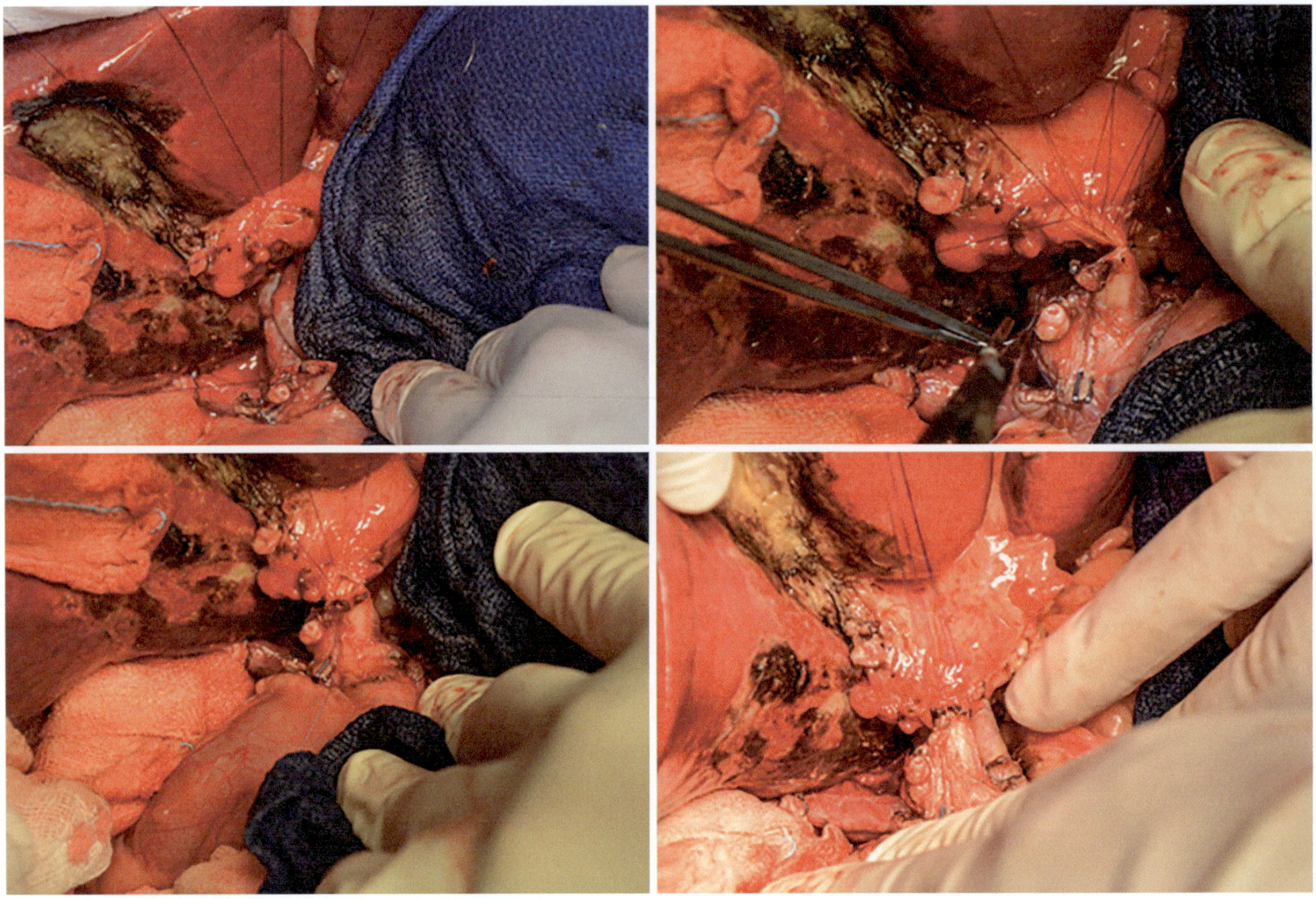

Fig. 4.19 Bile duct anastomosis

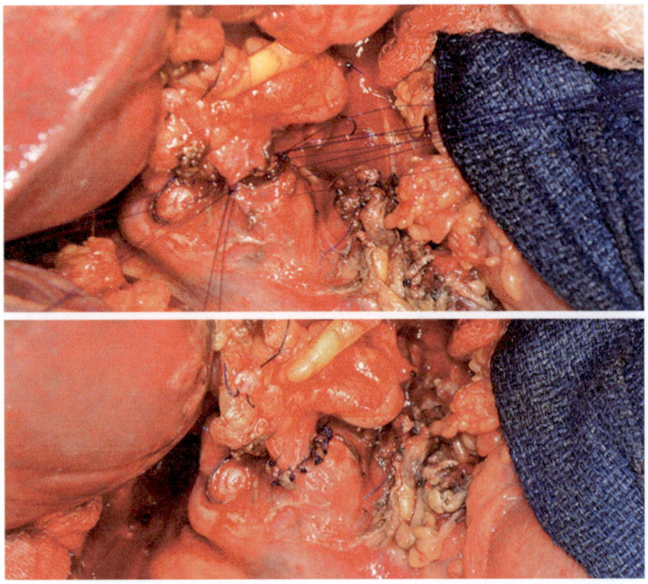

Fig. 4.20 Bile duct anastomosis

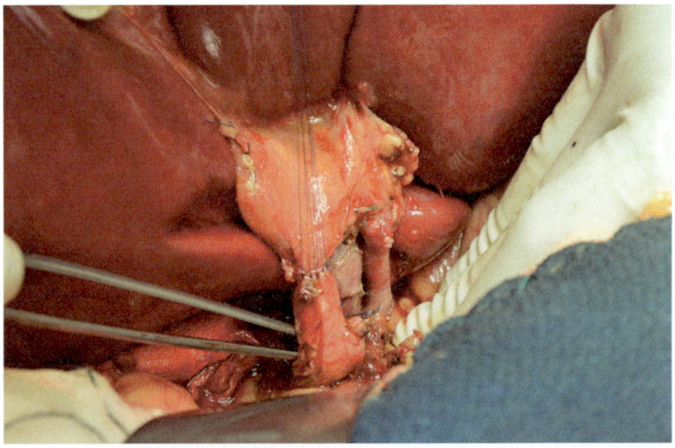

Fig. 4.21 Bile duct anastomosis

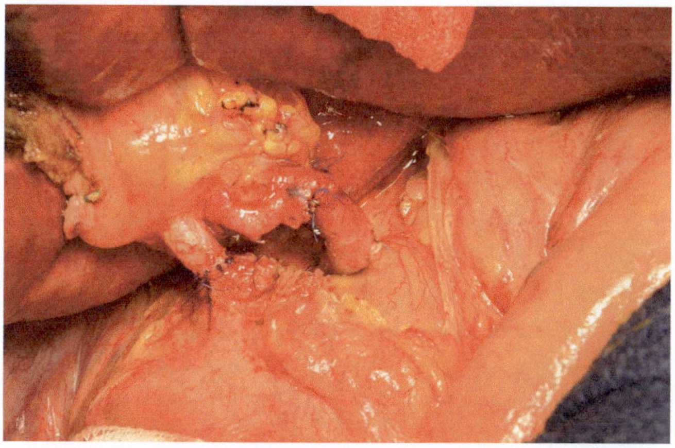

Fig. 4.22 Bile duct anastomosis

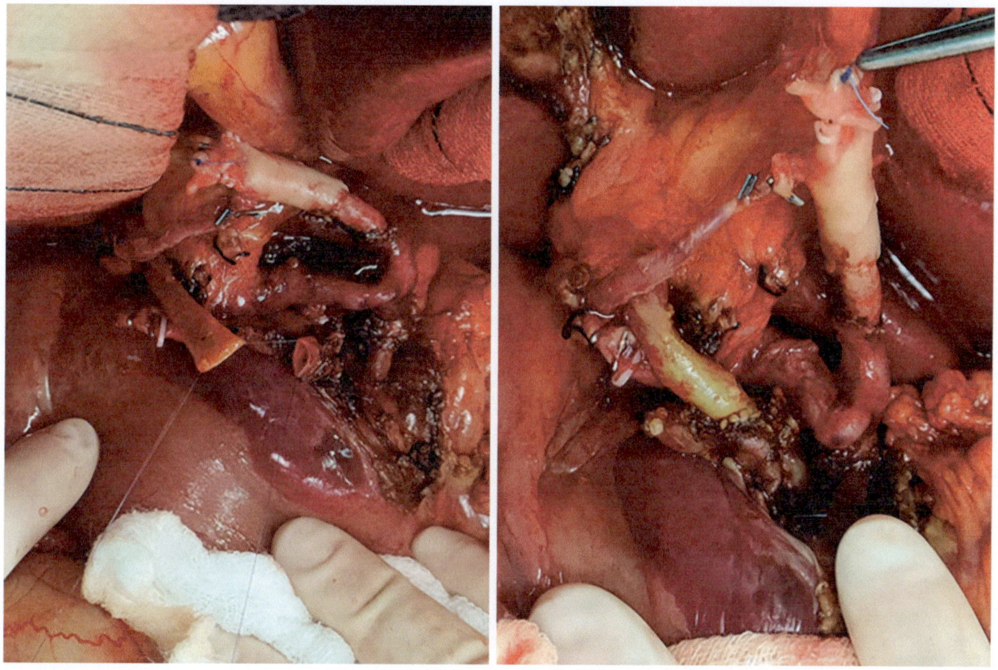

Fig. 4.23 Bile duct anastomosis with a replaced right hepatic artery

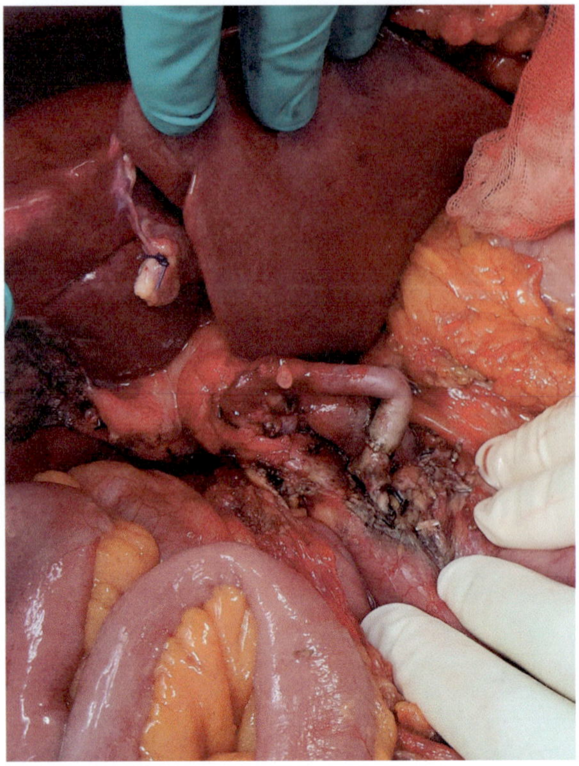

Fig. 4.24 Long graft hepatic artery

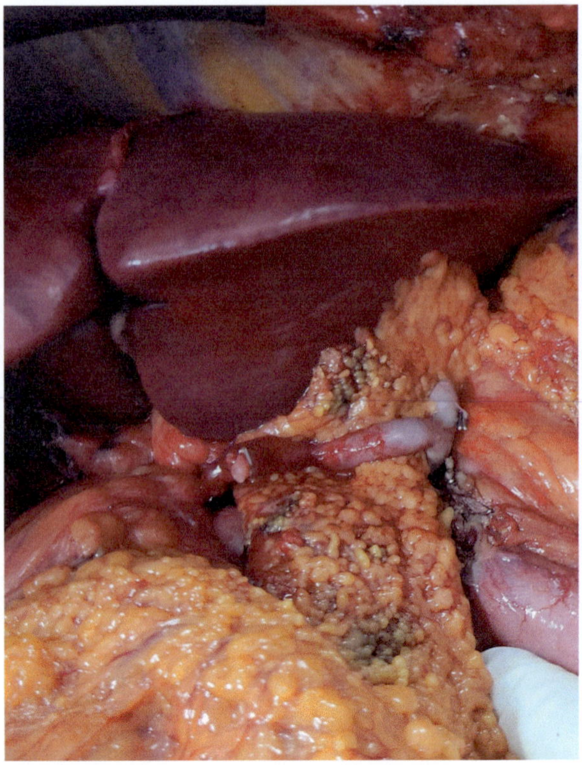

Fig. 4.25 Interposition of omental flap to prevent arterial kinking

Reference

1. Yilmaz S, Kutluturk K, Usta S, Akbulut S. Techniques of hepatic arterial reconstruction in liver transplantation. Langenbeck's Arch Surg. 2022;407(7):2607–18. https://doi.org/10.1007/s00423-022-02659-6. Epub 2022 Aug 26.

Complex Total Hepatectomy Including Inferior Vena Cava Resection

5

A complex liver transplantation is defined as a procedure in which recipient hepatectomy and/or graft implantation is anticipated to be technically difficult [1–3]. Piggyback total hepatectomy technique may be completely changed to total hepatectomy including the inferior vena cava resection because of technical complexity caused by the hypertrophied caudate lobe, severe inflammatory adhesion, and enlarged venous collaterals caused by portal hypertension. The use of veno-venous bypass may be necessary. Sclerosing encapsulating peritonitis, portal vein thrombosis, polycystic liver disease, and the presence of a previous bilio-enteric anastomosis or liver retransplantation are factors that increase the surgical difficulty (Figs. 5.1, 5.2, 5.3, 5.4, 5.5, 5.6, 5.7, 5.8, 5.9, 5.10, 5.11, 5.12, 5.13, 5.14, 5.15, 5.16, 5.17, 5.18, 5.19, 5.20, 5.21, 5.22, 5.23, 5.24, 5.25, 5.26, 5.27, and 5.28).

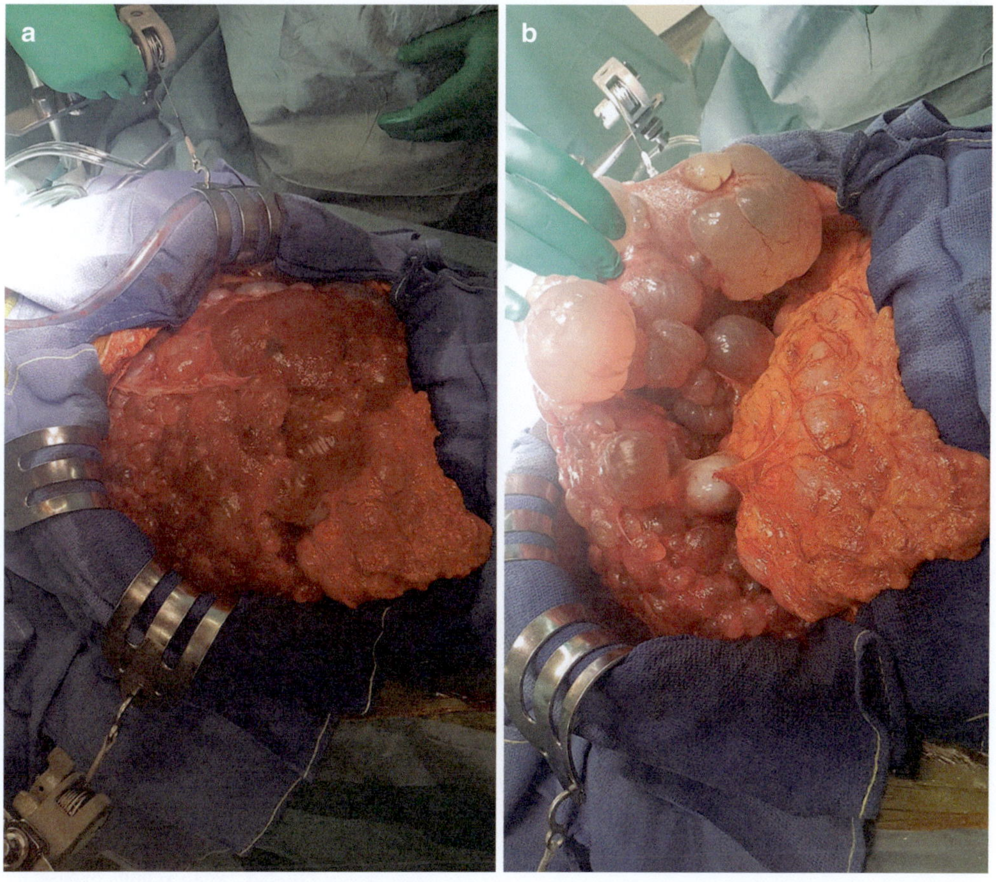

Fig. 5.1 Massive hepatomegaly related to polycystic liver disease as an example of difficult hepatectomy (**a**, **b**)

C. Lim et al., *Atlas of Liver Transplantation*, https://doi.org/10.1007/978-3-031-85264-0_5

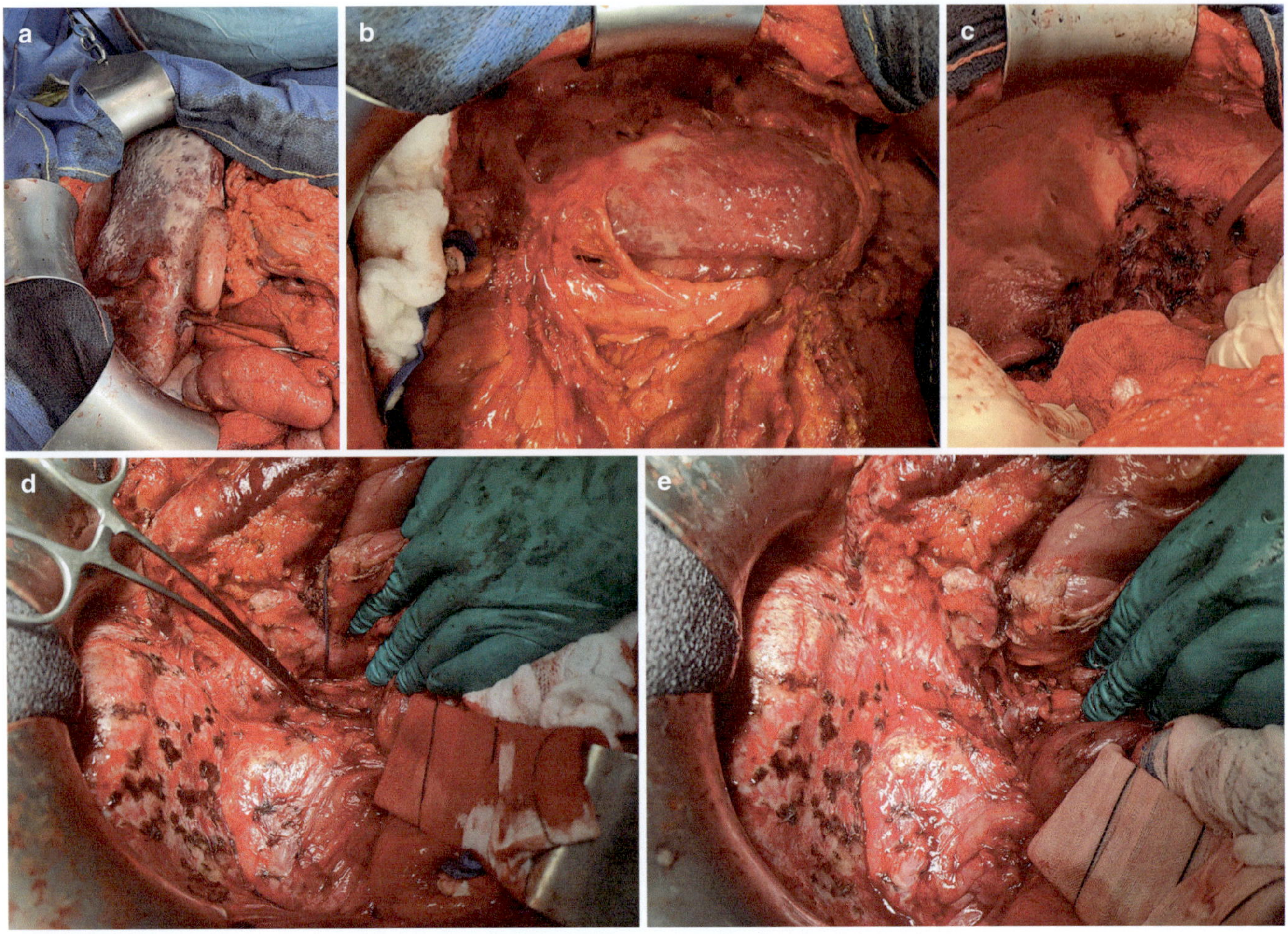

Fig. 5.2 Sclerosing encapsulating peritonitis (the so-called cocoon abdomen). (**a–c**) The native liver and the diaphragm are covered with a thick fibrotic peel. (**d**) Complex piggyback total hepatectomy in the presence of sclerosing encapsulating peritonitis. (**e**) Portocaval shunt performed after total hepatectomy

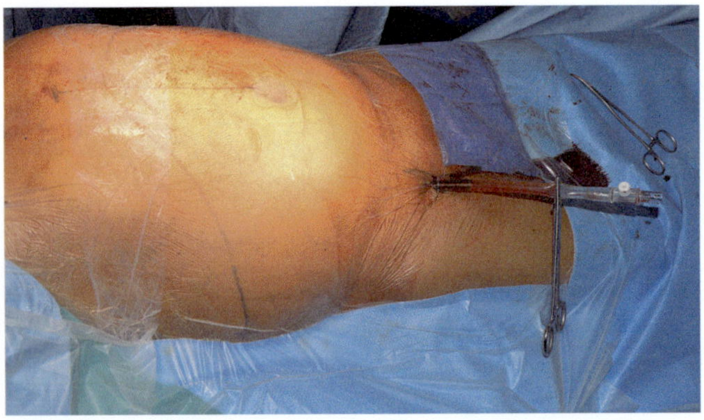

Fig. 5.3 Veno-venous bypass: right femoral vein cannulation

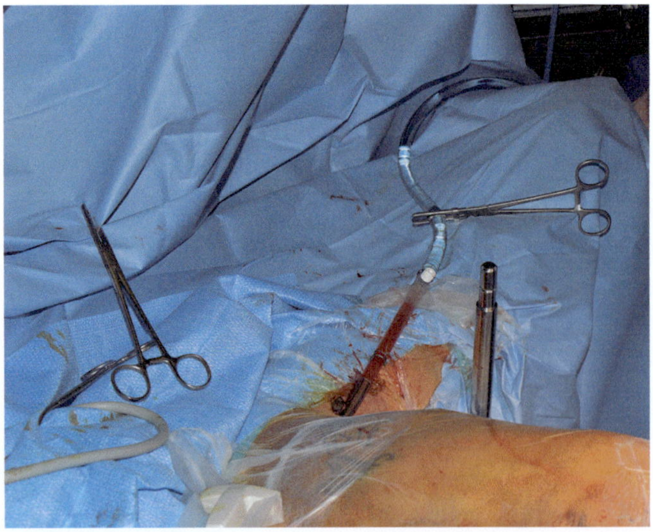

Fig. 5.4 Veno-venous bypass: left axillary vein cannulation

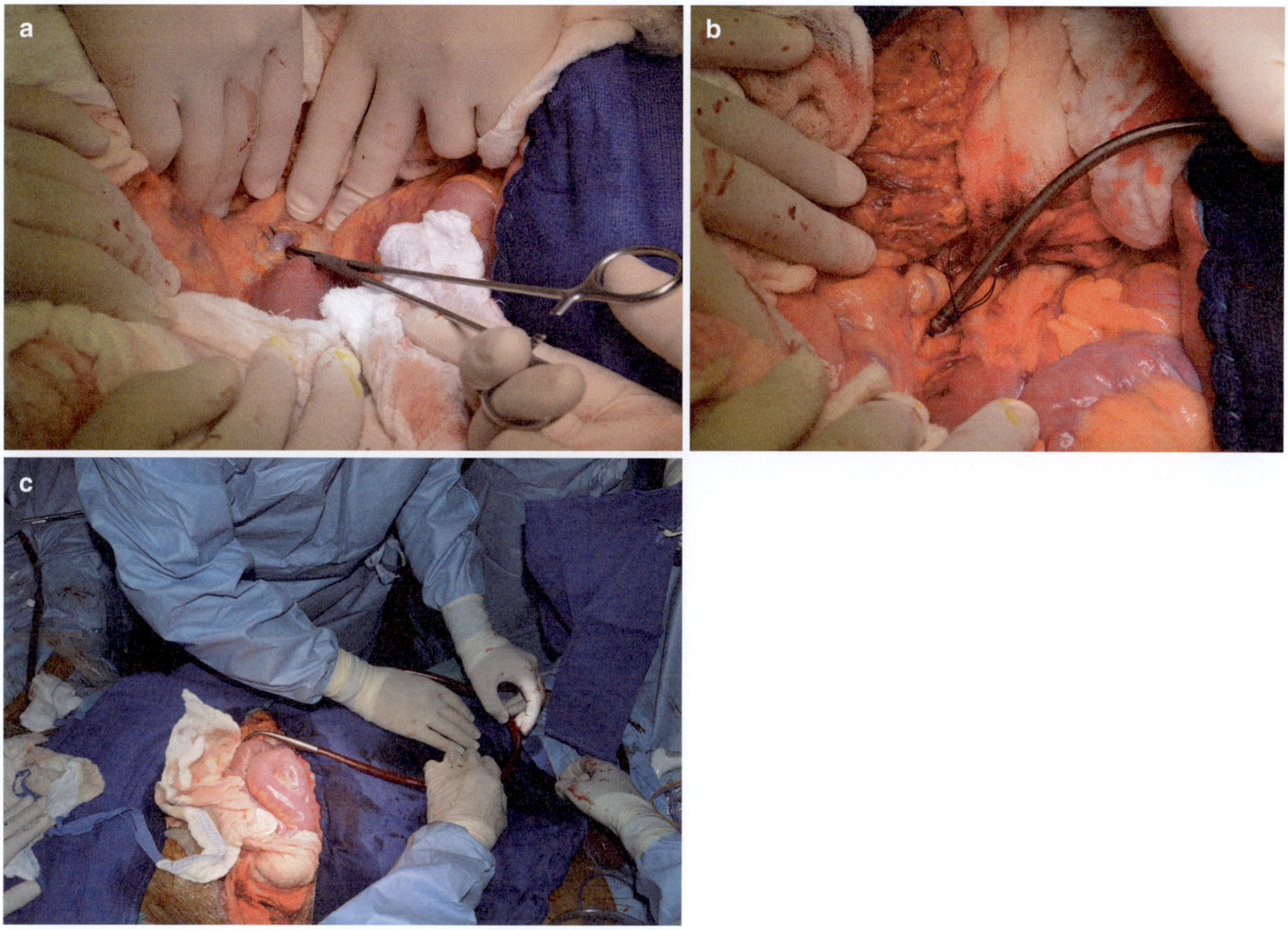

Fig. 5.5 Veno-venous bypass: inferior mesenteric vein cannulation (**a–c**)

Fig. 5.6 Veno-venous bypass: umbilical vein cannulation (**a**, **b**)

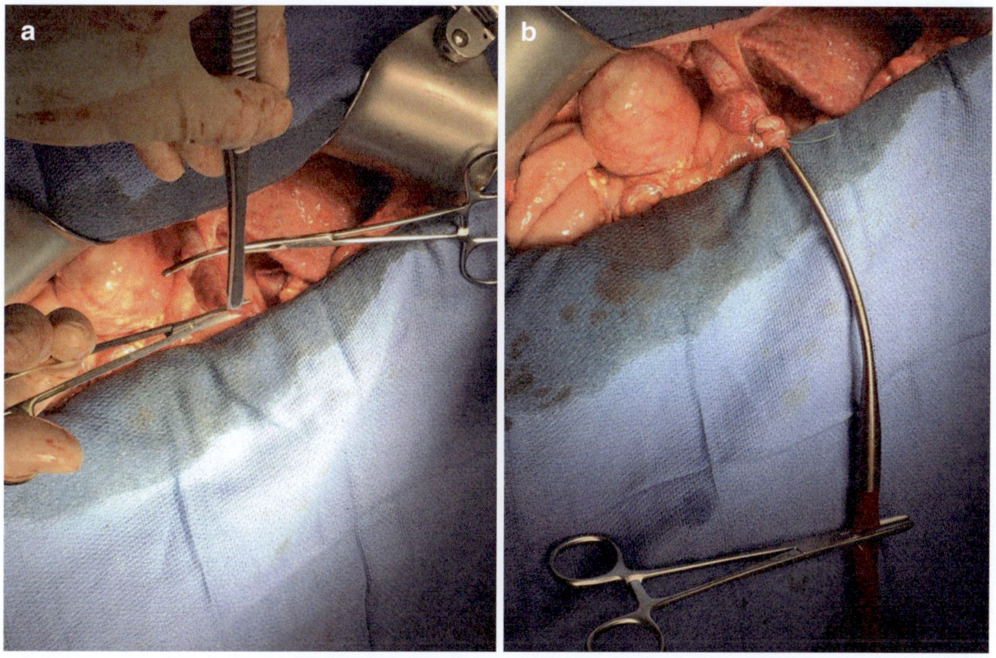

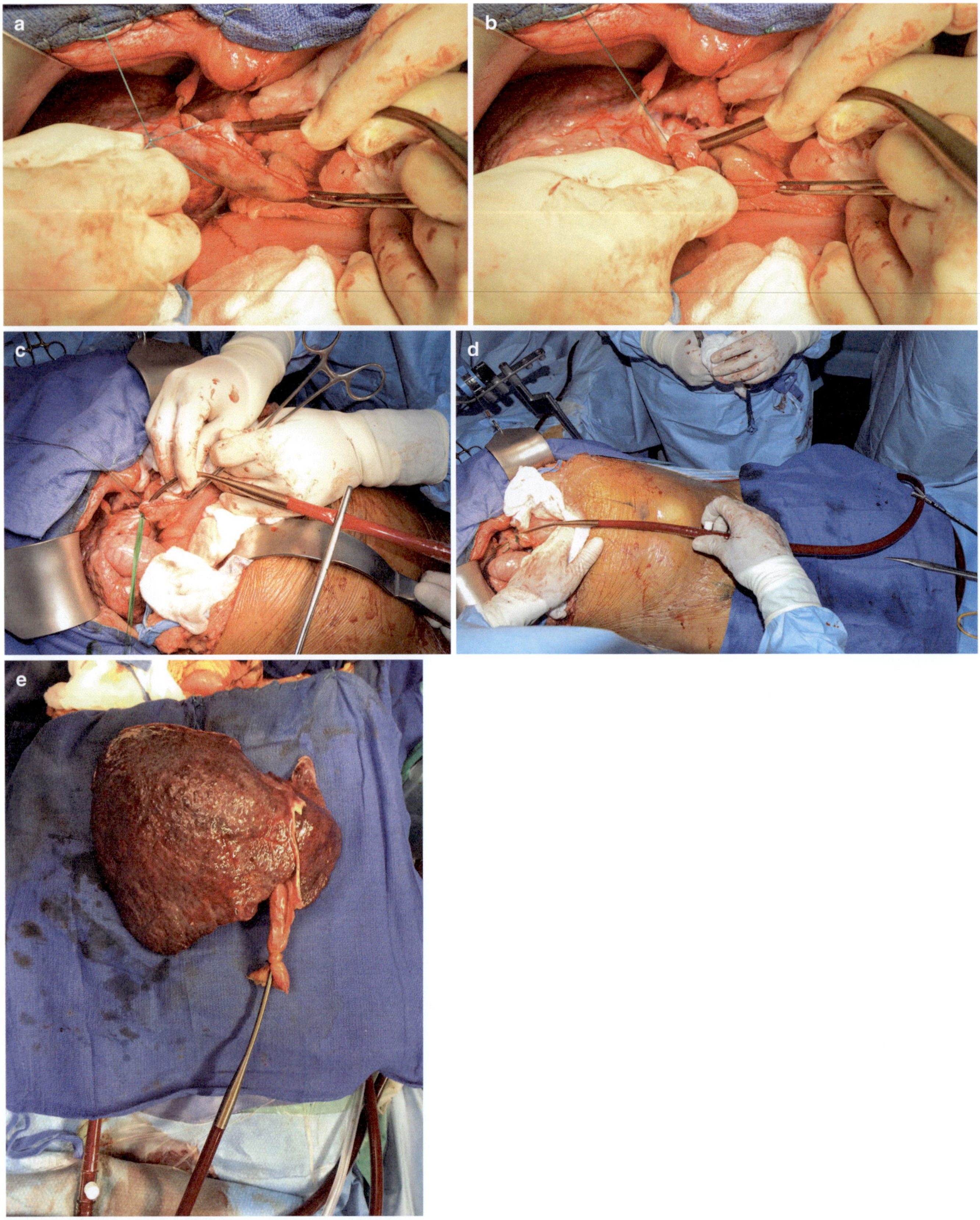

Fig. 5.7 Veno-venous bypass: umbilical vein cannulation (**a**–**e**)

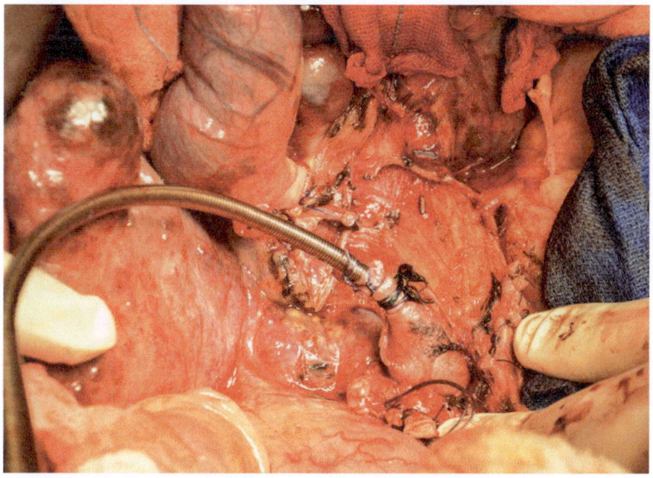

Fig. 5.8 Veno-venous bypass: portal vein cannulation

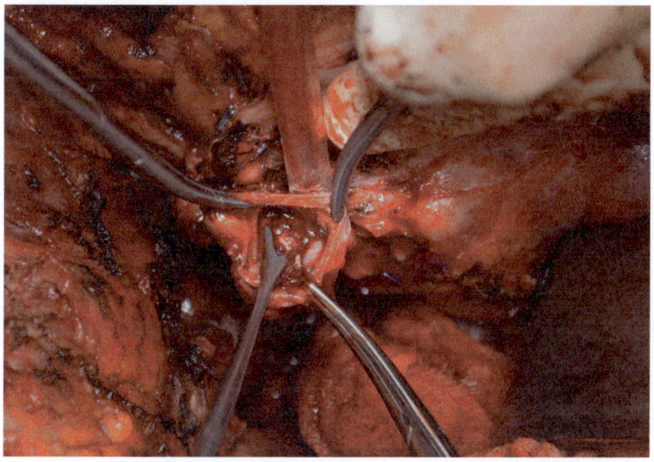

Fig. 5.9 Partial portal vein thrombosis

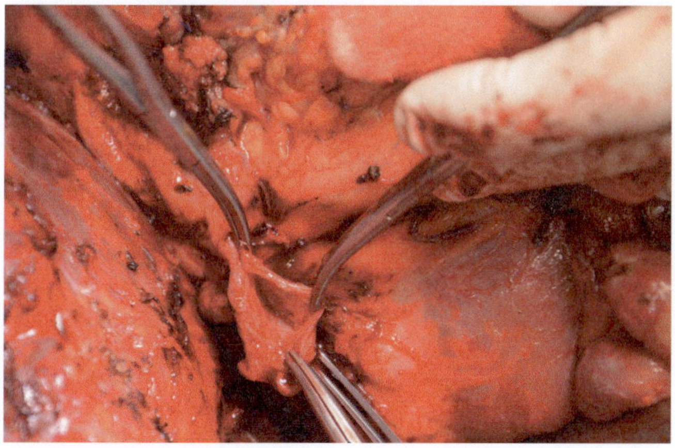

Fig. 5.10 Portal vein after thrombectomy

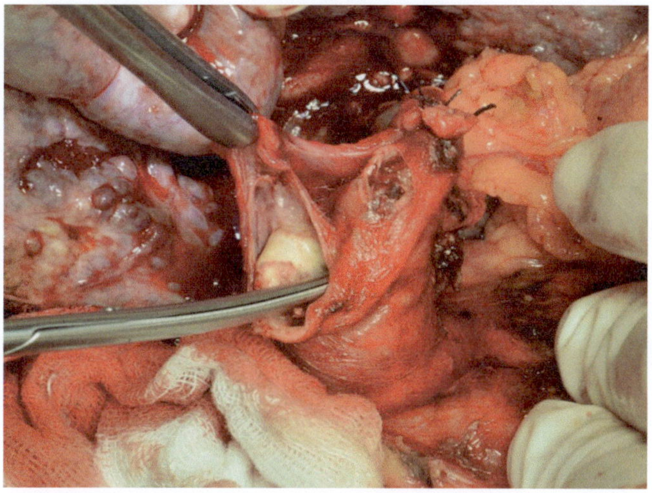

Fig. 5.11 Complete portal vein thrombosis

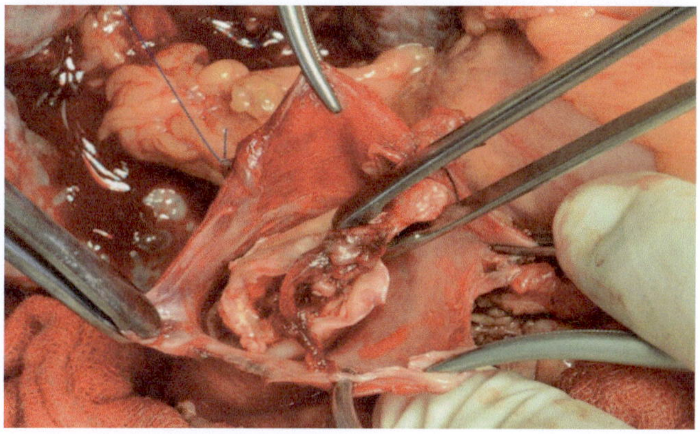

Fig. 5.12 Portal vein thrombectomy

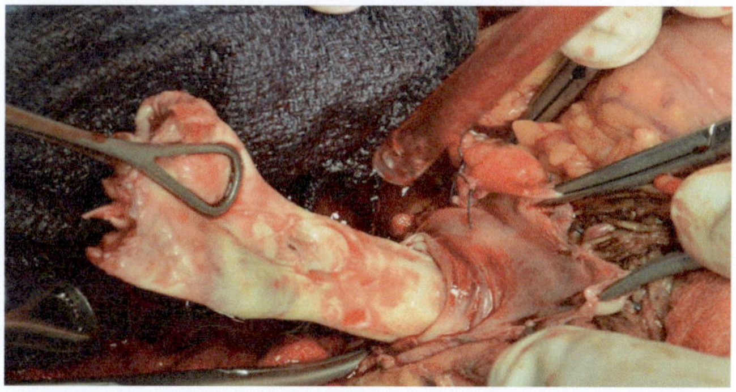

Fig. 5.13 Portal vein thrombectomy

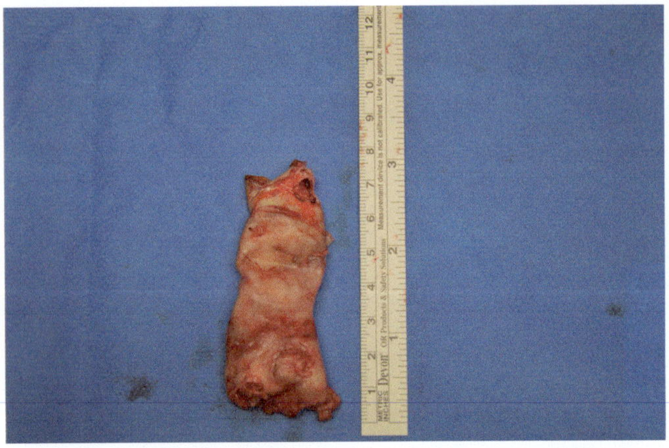

Fig. 5.14 Portal vein thrombus

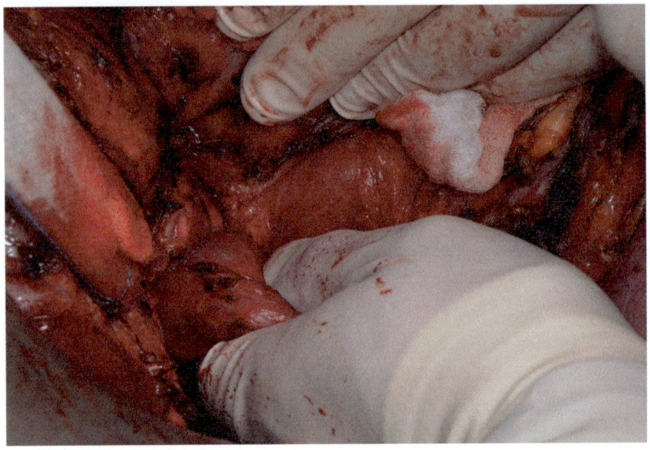

Fig. 5.15 Dissection of the bilio-enteric anastomosis

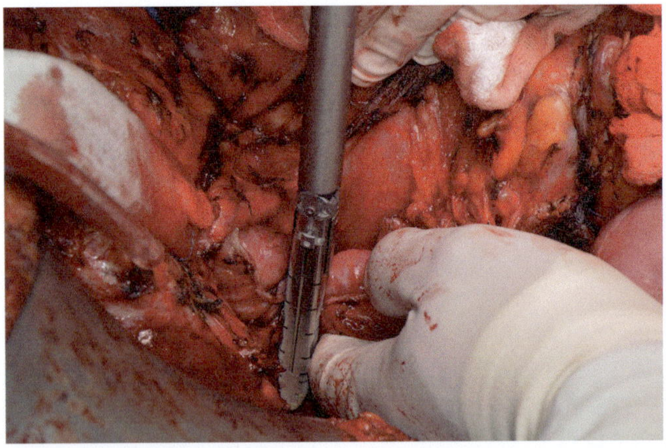

Fig. 5.16 Section of the bilio-enteric anastomosis using a vascular stapler

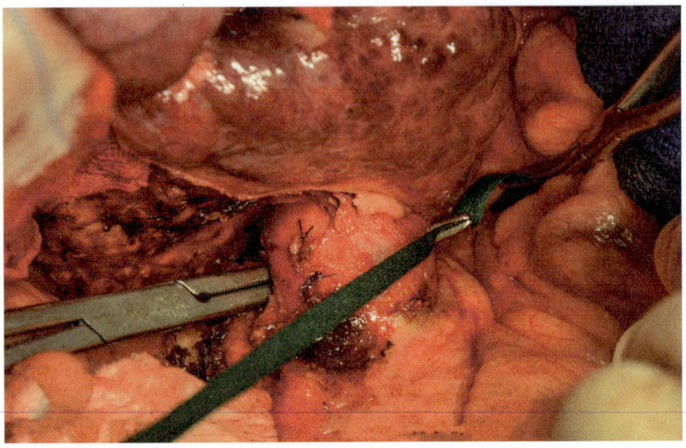

Fig. 5.17 Vascular exclusion of the liver: control of the infrahepatic inferior vena cava

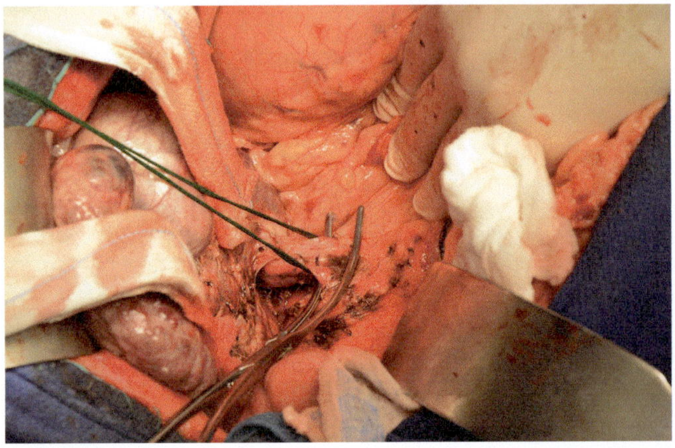

Fig. 5.18 Vascular exclusion of the liver: clamping of the infrahepatic inferior vena cava

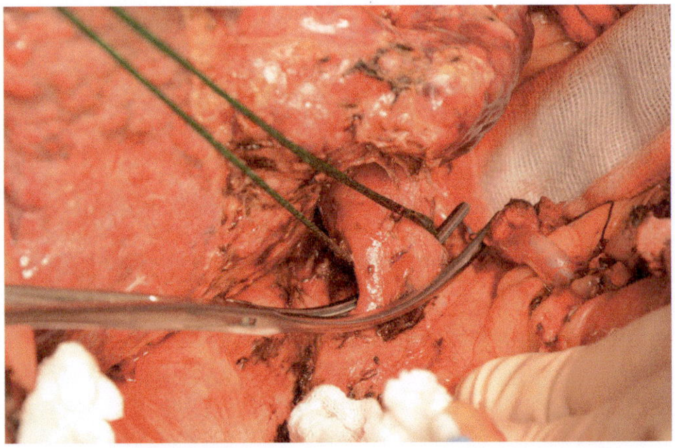

Fig. 5.19 Vascular exclusion of the liver: clamping of the infrahepatic inferior vena cava

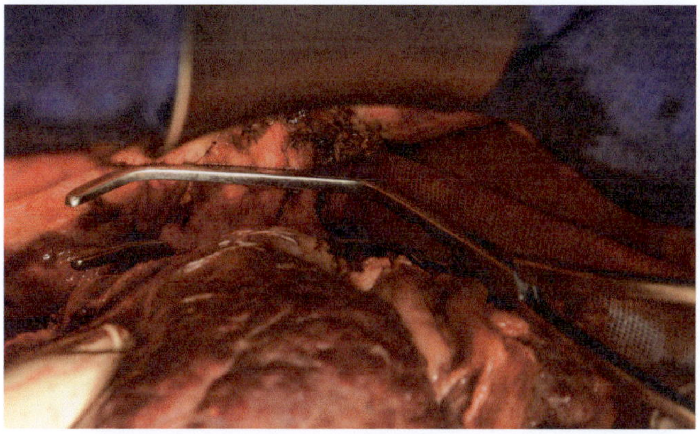

Fig. 5.20 Vascular exclusion of the liver: clamping of the suprahepatic inferior vena cava

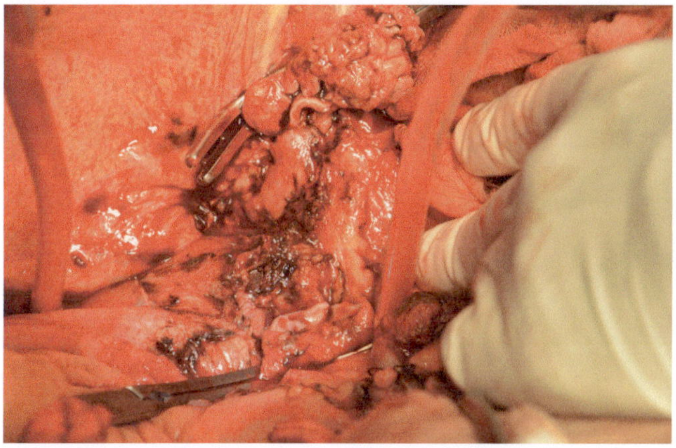

Fig. 5.21 Total hepatectomy including the native inferior vena cava resection

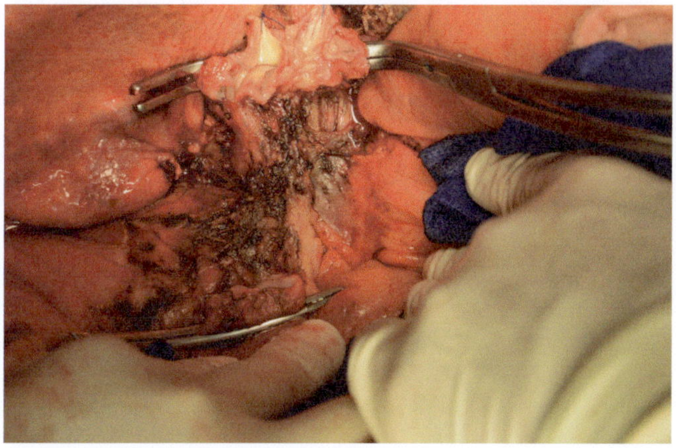

Fig. 5.22 Preparation of the suprahepatic inferior vena cava before caval anastomosis

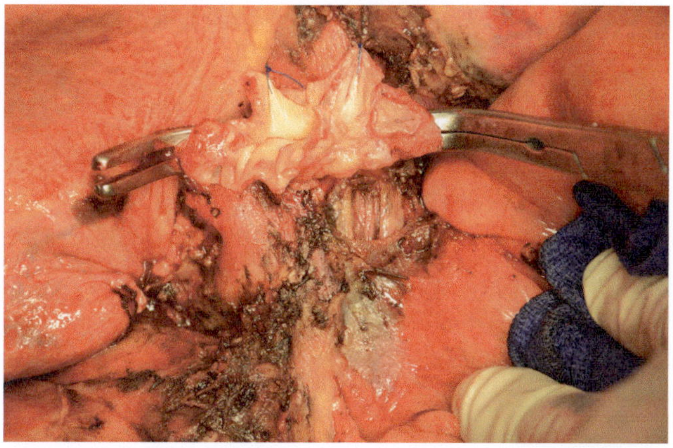

Fig. 5.23 Preparation of the anterior wall of the suprahepatic inferior vena cava

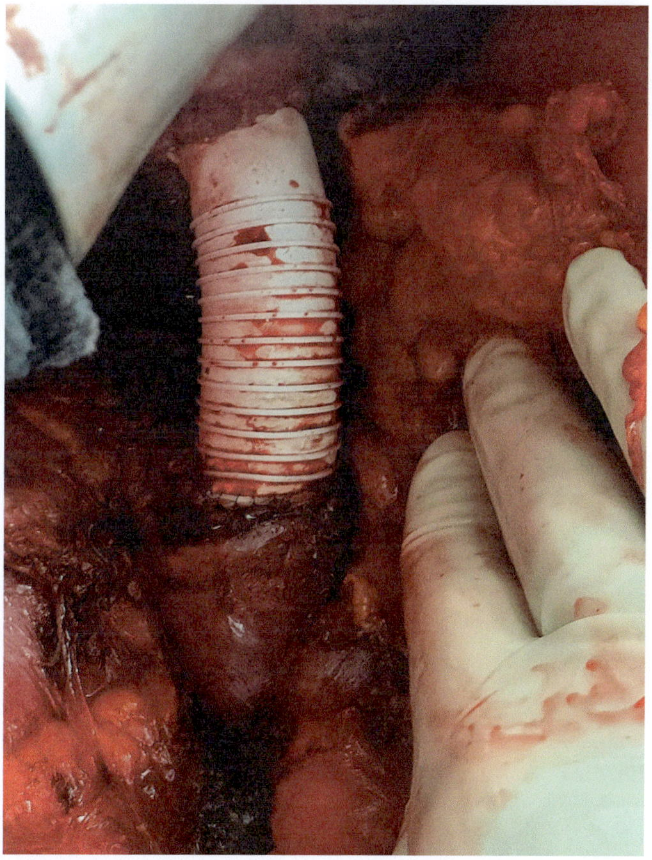

Fig. 5.24 A polytetrafluoroethylene (PTFE) graft was used for a cavo-caval shunt as an alternative technique to veno-venous bypass after total hepatectomy including the inferior vena cava resection

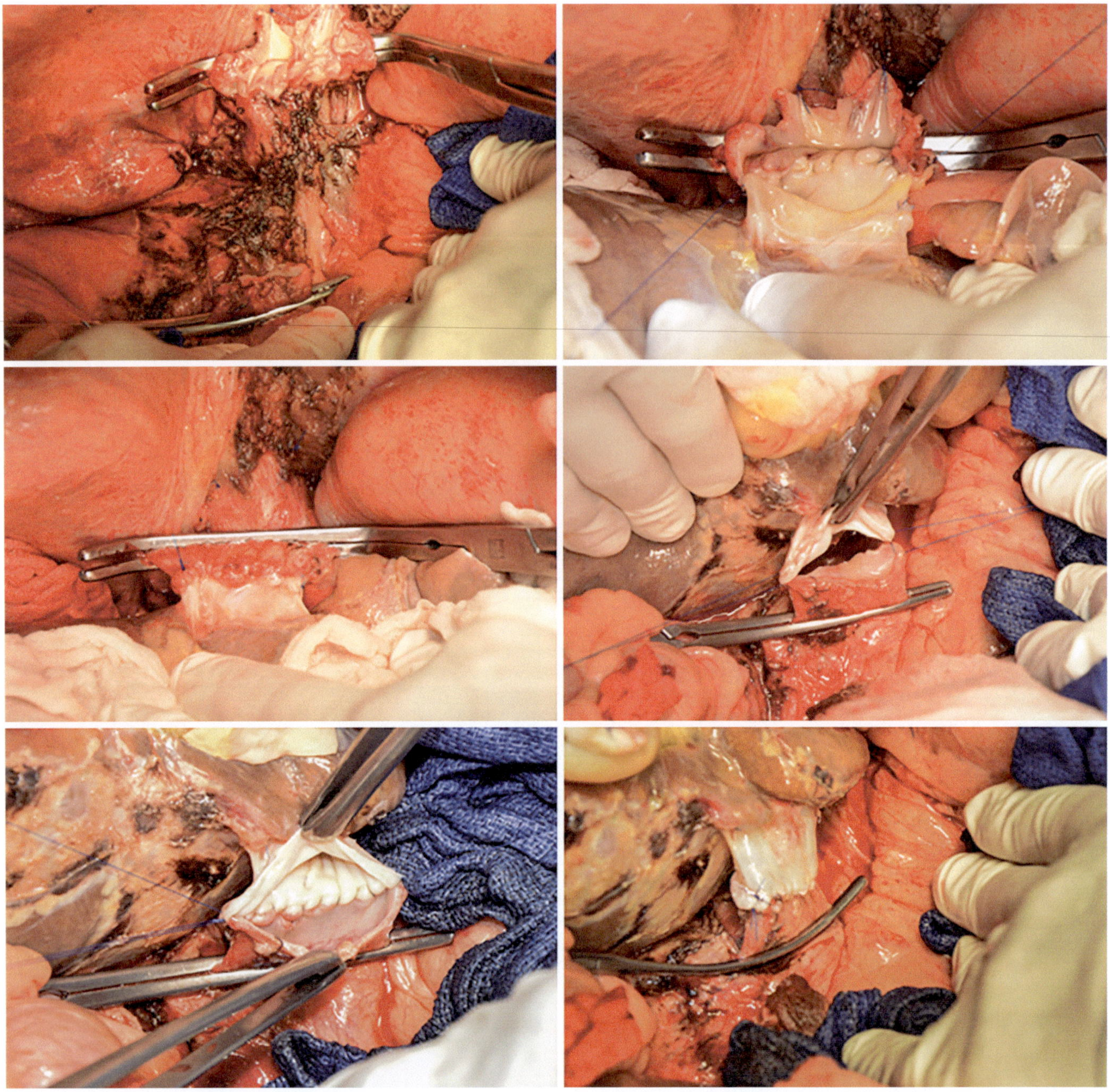

Fig. 5.25 Graft implantation starting with the suprahepatic inferior vena cava anastomosis followed by the infrahepatic inferior vena cava anastomosis

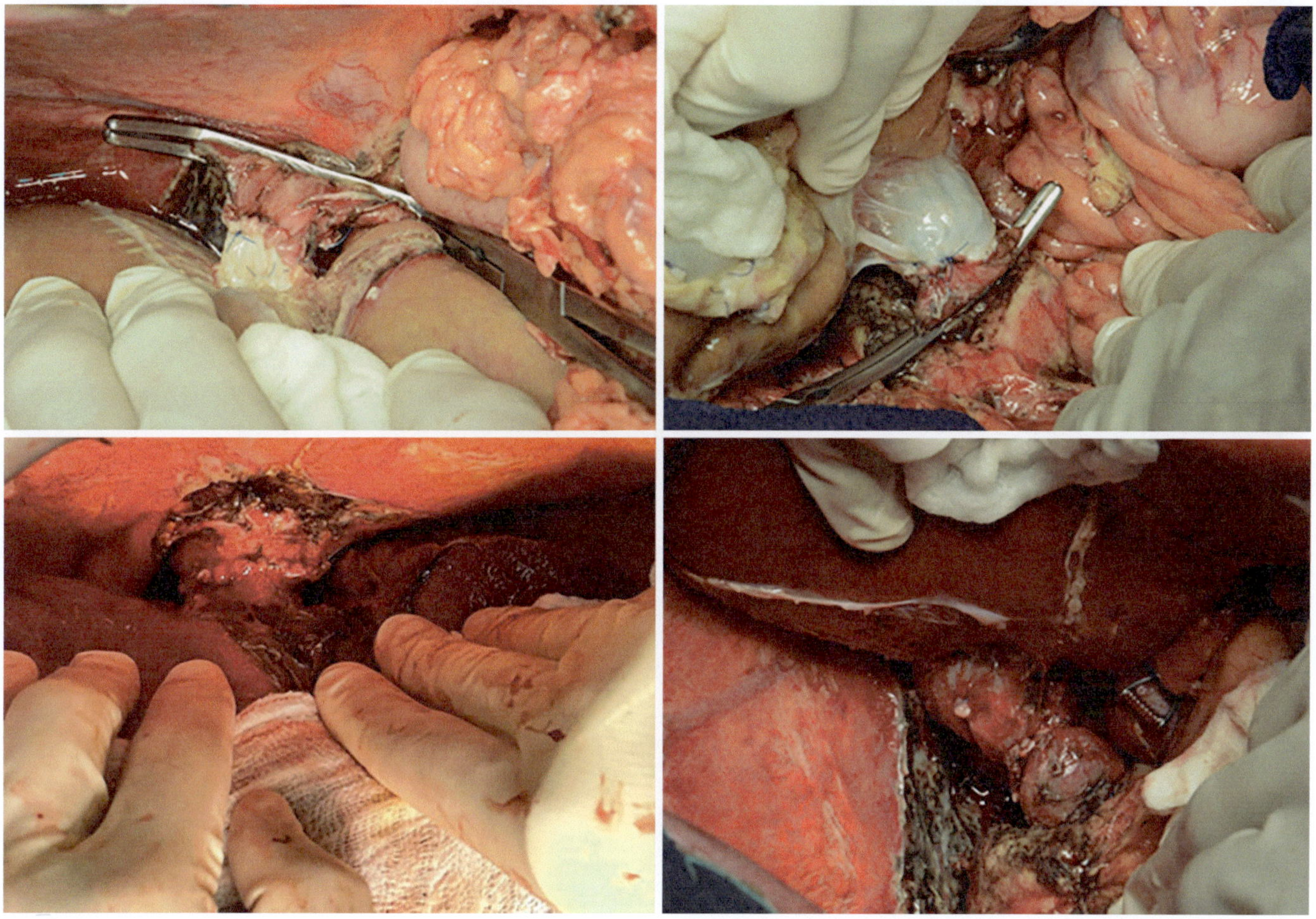

Fig. 5.26 Clamping and unclamping of the supra- and infrahepatic inferior vena cava anastomoses

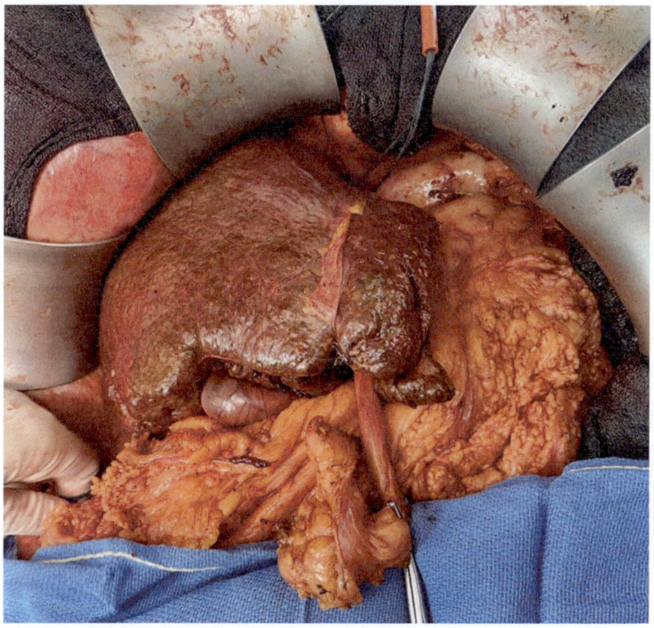

Fig. 5.27 The left lateral sectionectomy first approach during total hepatectomy (anterior view)

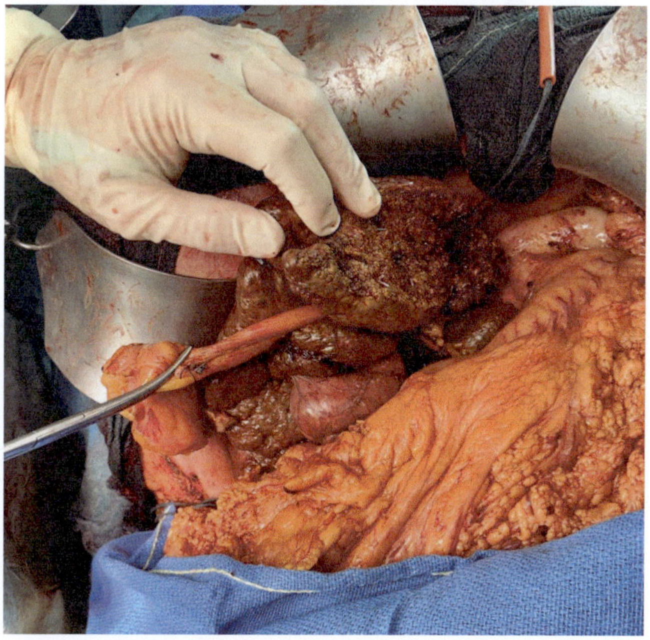

Fig. 5.28 The left lateral sectionectomy first approach during total hepatectomy (lateral view)

References

1. Azoulay D, Salloum C, Llado L, Ramos E, Lopez-Dominguez J, Cachero A, et al. Defining surgical difficulty of liver transplantation. Ann Surg. 2023;277(1):144–50. https://doi.org/10.1097/SLA.0000000000005017. Epub 2021 Jun 18.
2. Lim C, Turco C, Goumard C, Jeune F, Perdigao F, Savier E, et al. Perceptions of surgical difficulty in liver transplantation: a European survey and development of the Pitie-Salpetriere classification. Surgery. 2023;174(4):979–93. https://doi.org/10.1016/j.surg.2023.06.041. Epub 2023 Aug 4.
3. Sommier L, Lim C, Jeune F, Goumard C, Turco C, Salloum C, et al. European validation of the classification for the anticipated difficulty of liver transplantation. HPB (Oxford). 2024;26(8):1033–9. https://doi.org/10.1016/j.hpb.2024.05.004. Epub 2024 May 15.

6 Portal Inflow Reconstruction for Complex Portal Vein Thrombosis

Non-tumoral portal vein thrombosis is present at the time of liver transplantation in 5–26% of cirrhotic patients. The prevalence of complex portal vein thrombosis has been reported in 2.2% [1]. Portal inflow reconstruction is defined as non-physiological when porto-portal anastomosis could not be performed. In addition to porto-portal anastomosis, the reconstruction of portal flow is physiological when the splanchnic venous blood from a large portosystemic shunt (spontaneous or surgical) can be directed to the graft, either by anastomosis of the shunt to the graft portal vein or anastomosis of the tributary of the inferior vena cava (which drains this shunt) to the graft portal vein.

Physiological reconstructions include large left gastric vein to portal anastomosis and left renal vein to graft portal vein anastomosis (in patients with a spontaneous or surgical splenorenal shunt) (Figs. 6.1, 6.2, 6.3, 6.4, 6.5, 6.6, 6.7, 6.8, 6.9, 6.10, 6.11, 6.12, 6.13, 6.14, 6.15, 6.16, 6.17, 6.18, 6.19, 6.20, and 6.21).

C. Lim et al., *Atlas of Liver Transplantation*, https://doi.org/10.1007/978-3-031-85264-0_6

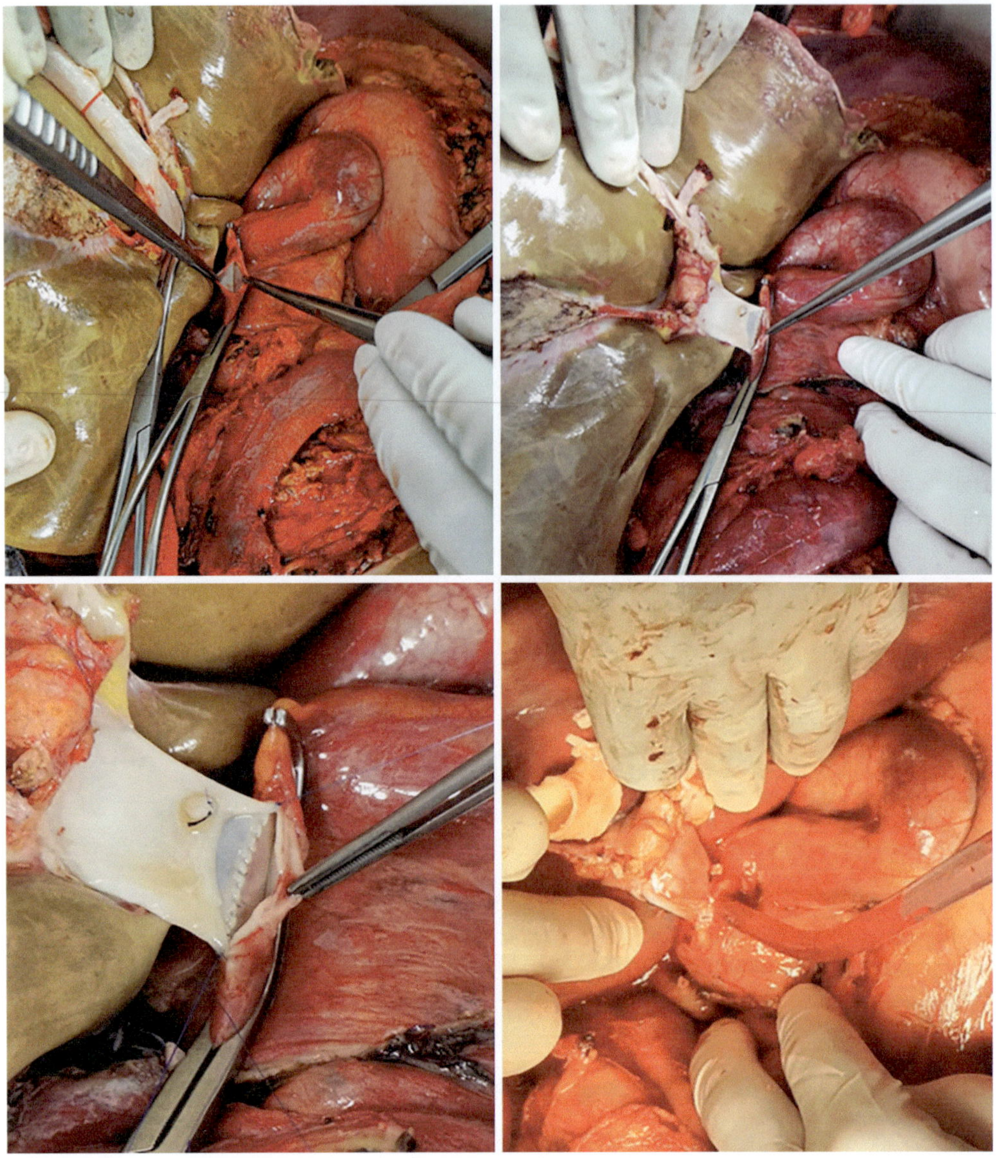

Fig. 6.1 Coronary-portal anastomosis. Lateral clamping of the large native left gastric vein using a Satinsky forceps. End-to-side anastomosis between the graft portal vein and the native left gastric vein

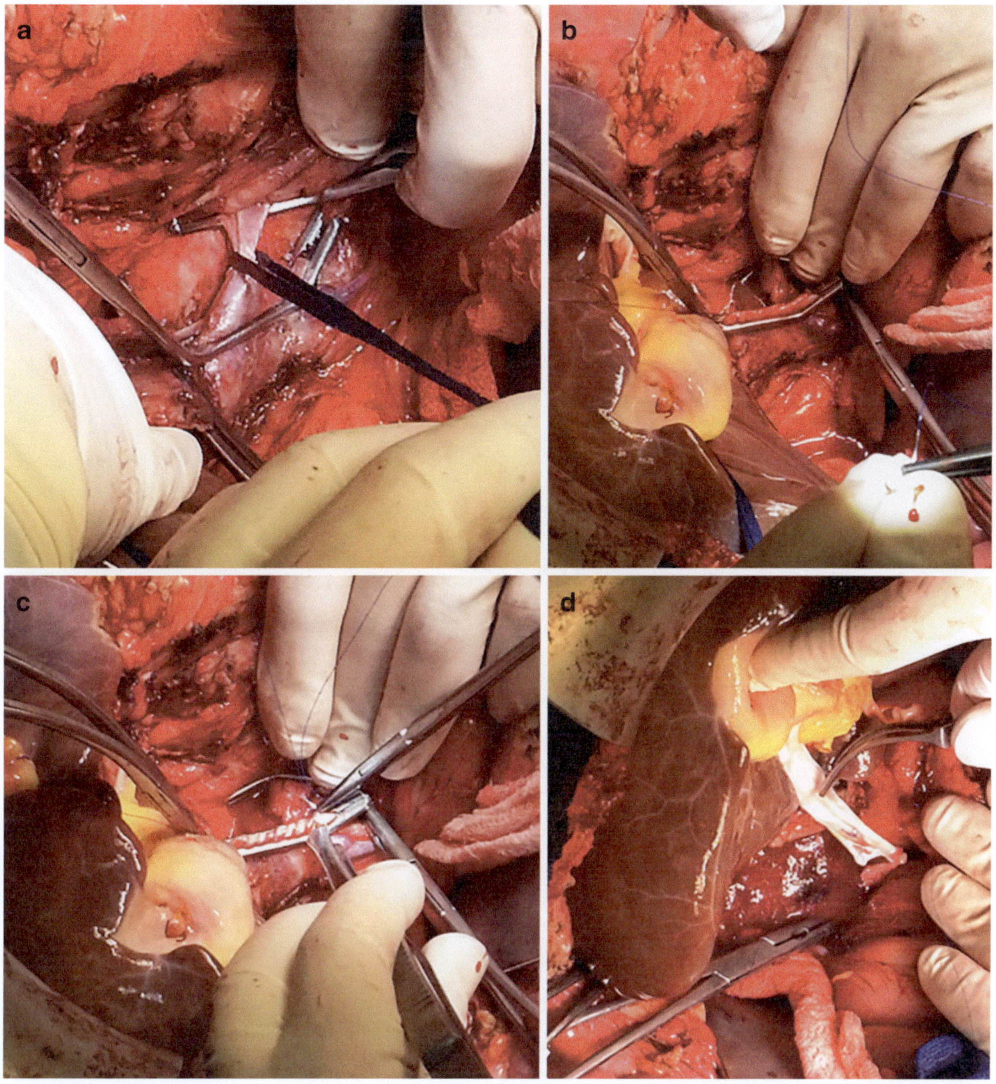

Fig. 6.2 Reno-portal anastomosis: (**a**) Lateral clamping of the inferior vena cava at the level of the left renal vein using a Satinsky forceps. (**b**) Section of the left renal vein. (**c**) Closure of the inferior vena cava. (**d**) End-to-side anastomosis between the graft portal vein and the native left renal vein

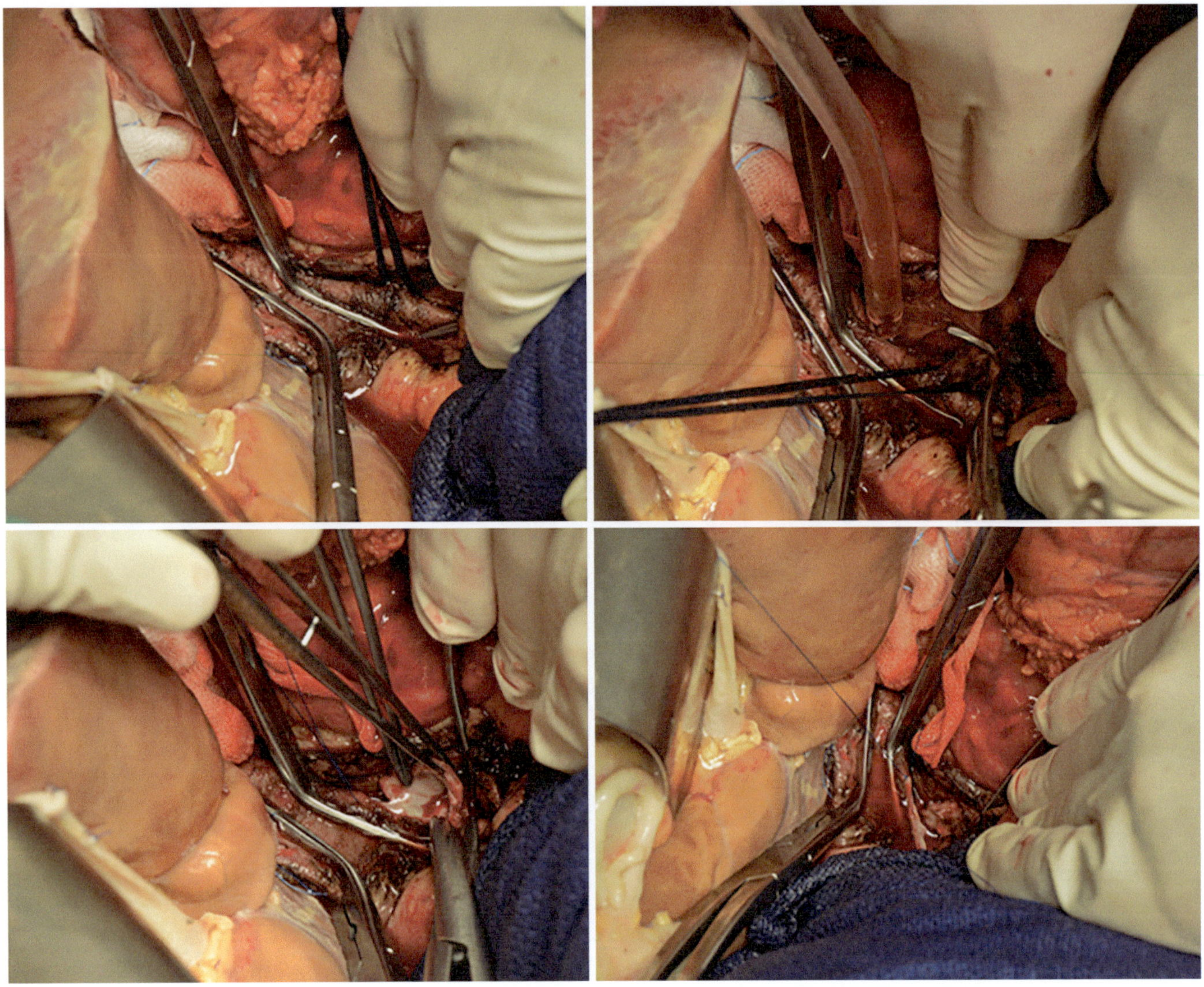

Fig. 6.3 Preparation of the left renal vein for a reno-portal anastomosis

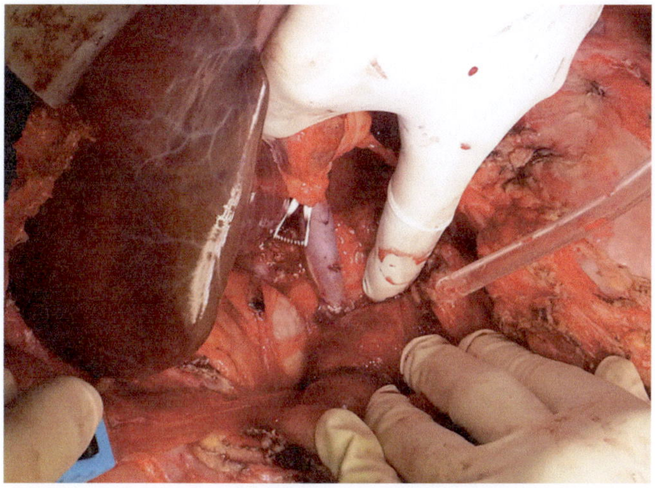

Fig. 6.4 Reno-portal anastomosis using an interposed femoral vein allograft

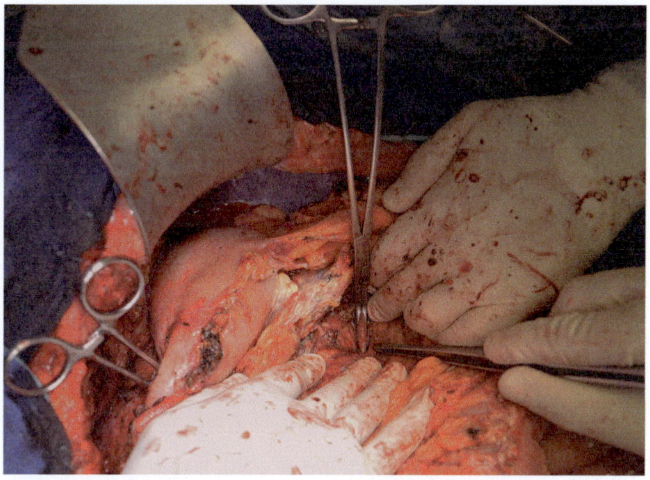

Fig. 6.6 A splenorenal shunt is performed in a patient with a reno-portal anastomosis without spontaneous splenorenal shunt. Lateral clamping of the left renal vein

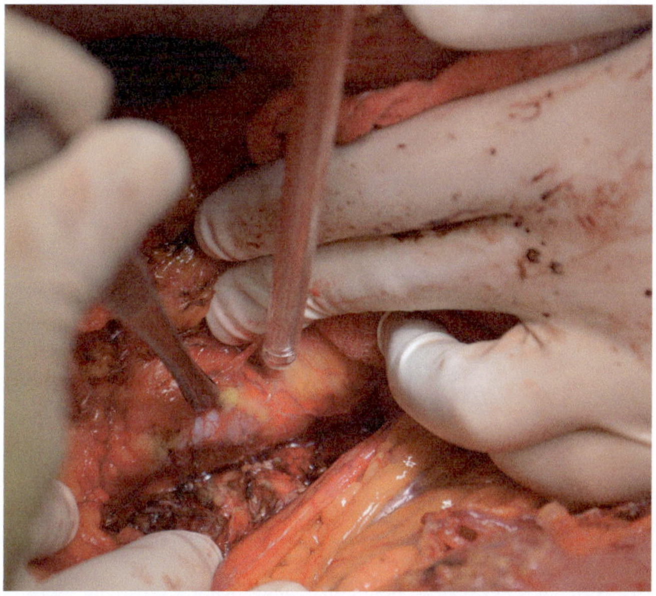

Fig. 6.5 A splenorenal shunt is performed in a patient with a reno-portal anastomosis without spontaneous splenorenal shunt. Dissection of the lateral aspect of the splenic vein

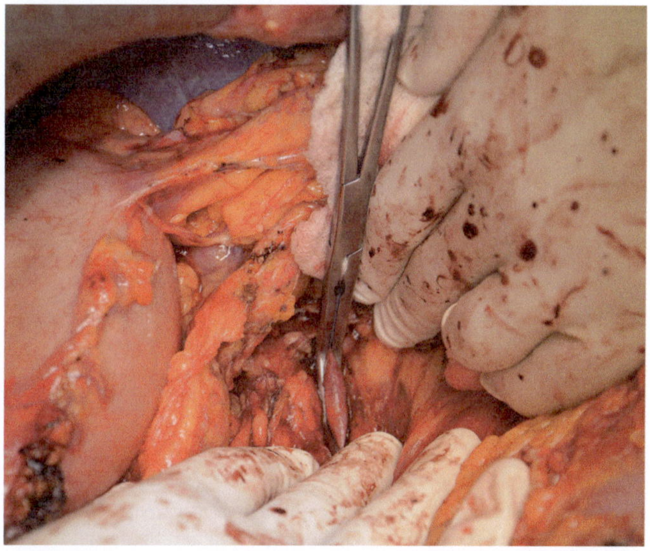

Fig. 6.7 A splenorenal shunt is performed in a patient with a reno-portal anastomosis without spontaneous splenorenal shunt. Lateral clamping of the left renal vein

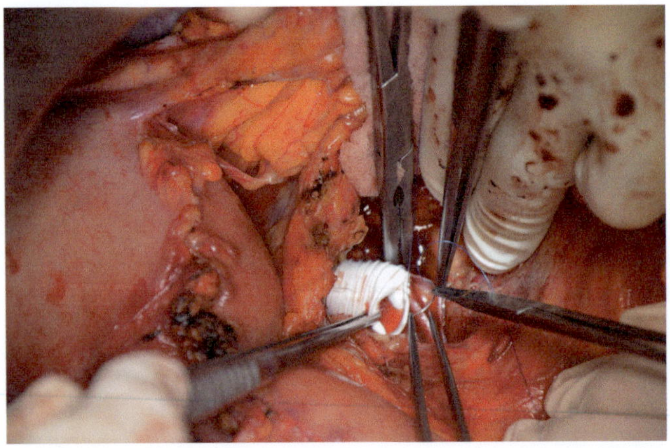

Fig. 6.8 A splenorenal shunt is performed in a patient with a reno-portal anastomosis without spontaneous splenorenal shunt. End-to-side anastomosis between the polytetrafluoroethylene (PTFE) graft and the left renal vein

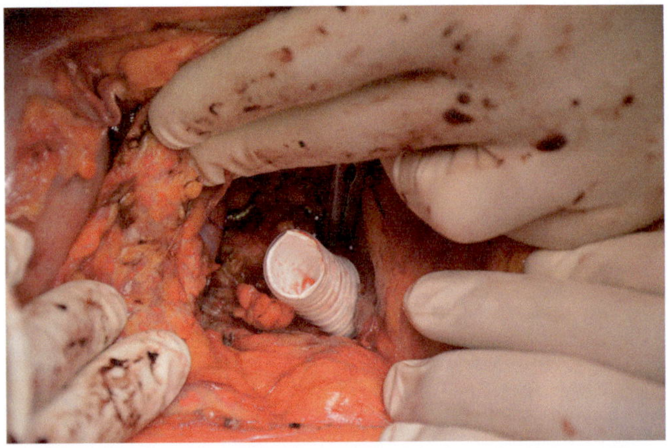

Fig. 6.9 A splenorenal shunt is performed in a patient with a reno-portal anastomosis without spontaneous splenorenal shunt. End-to-side anastomosis between the PTFE graft and the left renal vein

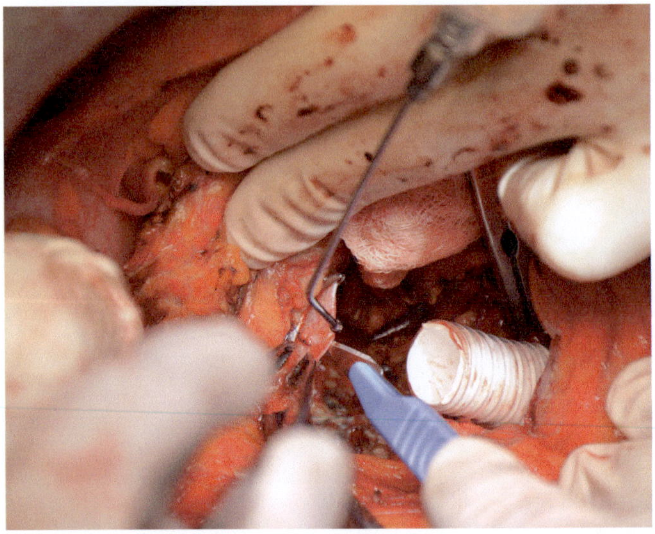

Fig. 6.10 A splenorenal shunt is performed in a patient with a reno-portal anastomosis without spontaneous splenorenal shunt. Incision of the wall of the native splenic vein

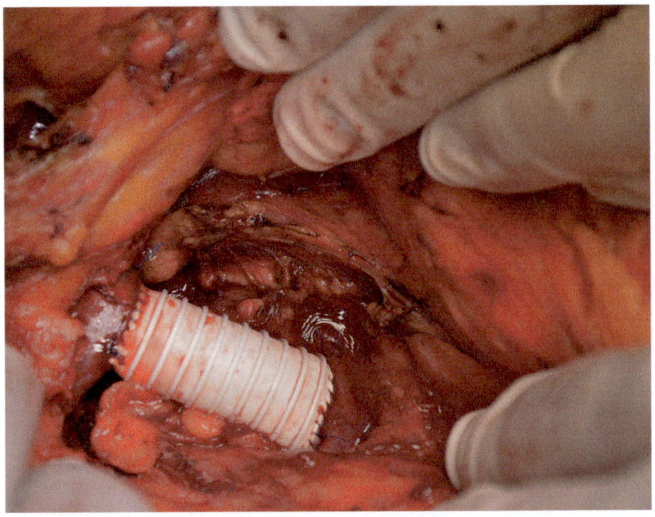

Fig. 6.11 A side-to-side splenorenal shunt using a prosthetic graft is performed in a patient with a reno-portal anastomosis without a spontaneous splenorenal shunt

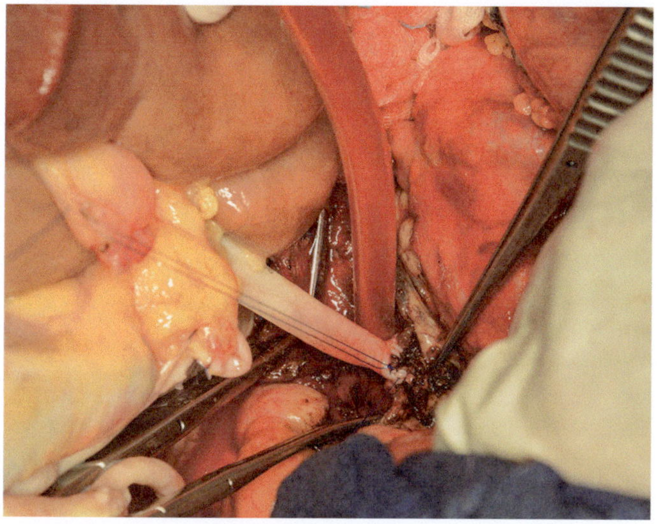

Fig. 6.12 A coronary-portal shunt is performed in a patient with a reno-portal anastomosis without spontaneous splenorenal shunt. Reno-portal anastomosis is first performed

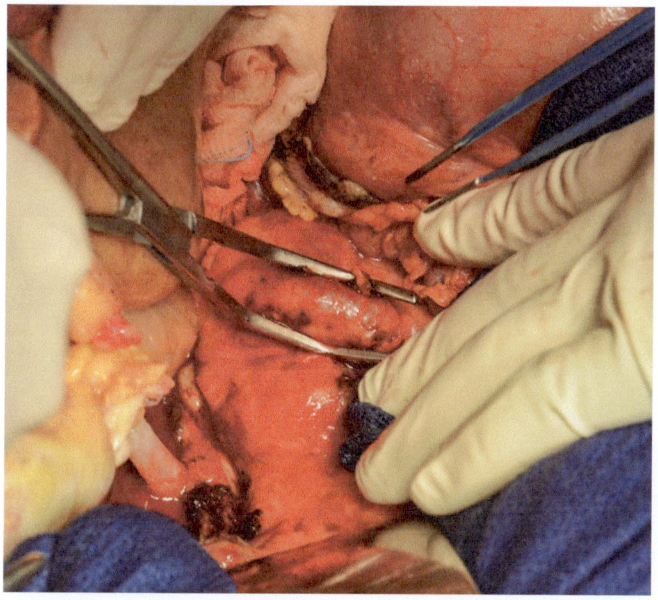

Fig. 6.13 A coronary-portal shunt is performed in a patient with a reno-portal anastomosis without spontaneous splenorenal shunt. Lateral clamping of the large left gastric vein

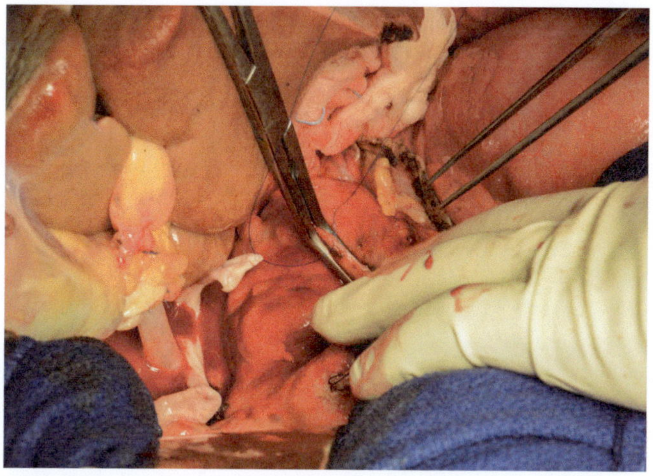

Fig. 6.14 A coronary-portal shunt is performed in a patient with a reno-portal anastomosis without spontaneous splenorenal shunt. Lateral clamping of the large left gastric vein

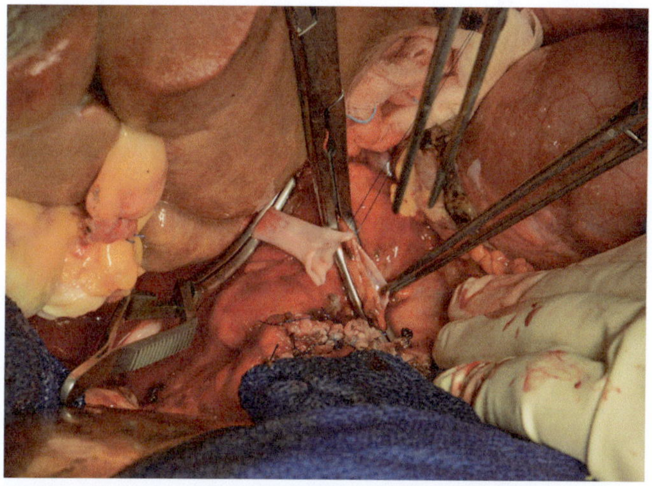

Fig. 6.15 A coronary-portal shunt is performed in a patient with a reno-portal anastomosis without spontaneous splenorenal shunt. End-to-side anastomosis between the venous allograft and the left gastric vein

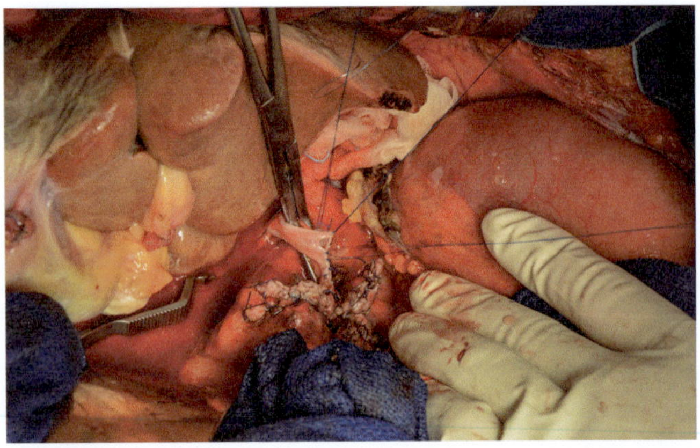

Fig. 6.16 A coronary-portal shunt is performed in a patient with a reno-portal anastomosis without spontaneous splenorenal shunt. End-to-side anastomosis between the venous allograft and the left gastric vein

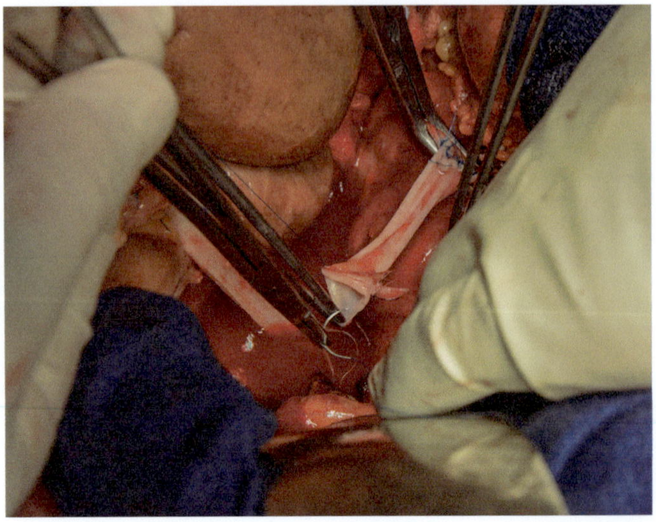

Fig. 6.18 A coronary-portal shunt is performed in a patient with a reno-portal anastomosis without spontaneous splenorenal shunt. End-to-side anastomosis between the venous allograft and the graft portal vein

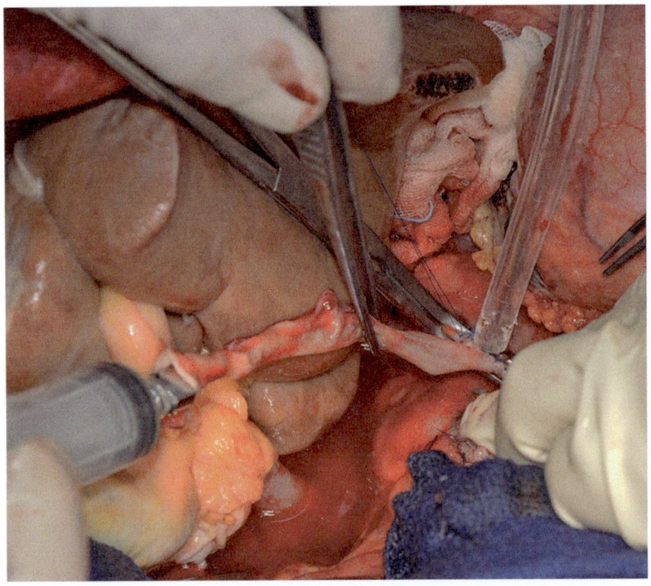

Fig. 6.17 A coronary-portal shunt is performed in a patient with a reno-portal anastomosis without spontaneous splenorenal shunt. End-to-side anastomosis between the venous allograft and the left gastric vein

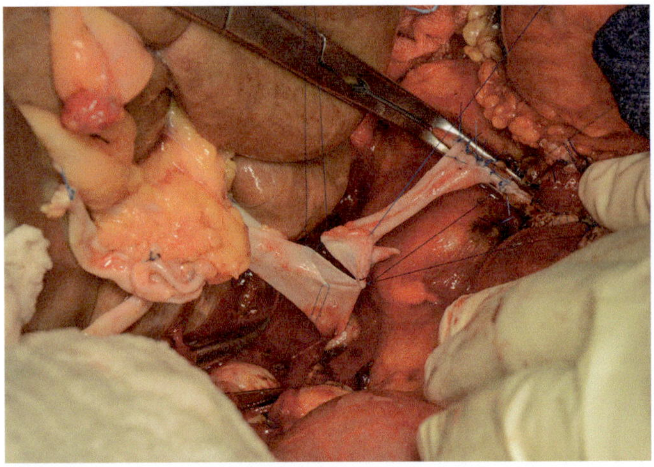

Fig. 6.19 A coronary-portal shunt is performed in a patient with a reno-portal anastomosis without spontaneous splenorenal shunt. End-to-side anastomosis between the venous allograft and the graft portal vein

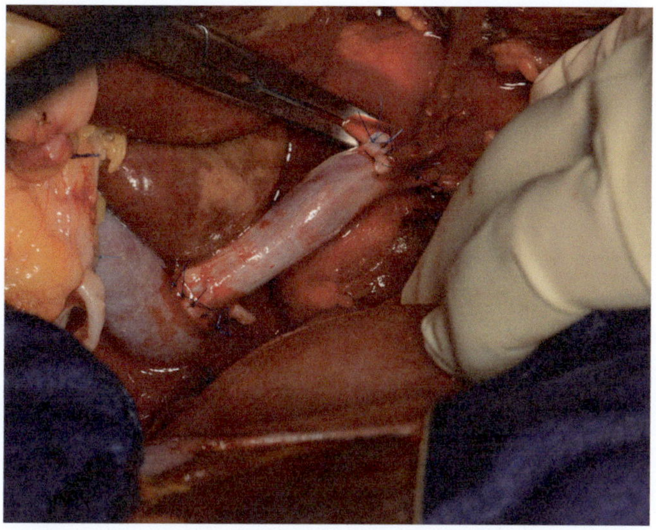

Fig. 6.20 A coronary-portal shunt is performed in a patient with a reno-portal anastomosis without spontaneous splenorenal shunt

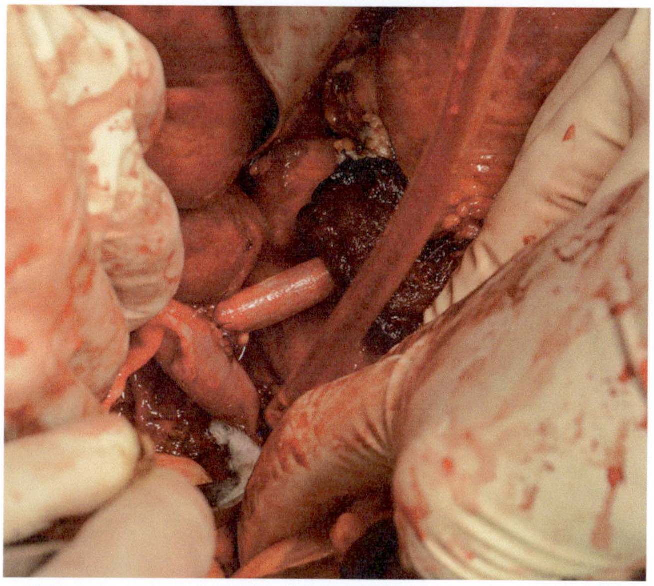

Fig. 6.21 A coronary-portal shunt is performed in a patient with a reno-portal anastomosis without spontaneous splenorenal shunt

Reference

1. Bhangui P, Lim C, Levesque E, et al. Novel classification of non-malignant portal vein thrombosis: a guide to surgical decision-making during liver transplantation. J Hepatol. 2019;71:1038–50.

7 Alternative Arterial Reconstructions

Standard arterial reconstruction is defined by graft hepatic artery to native hepatic artery anastomosis [1]. Other alternative arterial revascularization techniques include the recipient splenic artery, renal artery, and arterial conduits, which serve as interposition grafts implanted into the recipient supraceliac or infrarenal abdominal aorta and anastomosed to the donor hepatic artery (Figs. 7.1, 7.2, 7.3, 7.4, 7.5, 7.6, 7.7, 7.8, 7.9, 7.10, 7.11, 7.12, 7.13, and 7.14).

C. Lim et al., *Atlas of Liver Transplantation*, https://doi.org/10.1007/978-3-031-85264-0_7

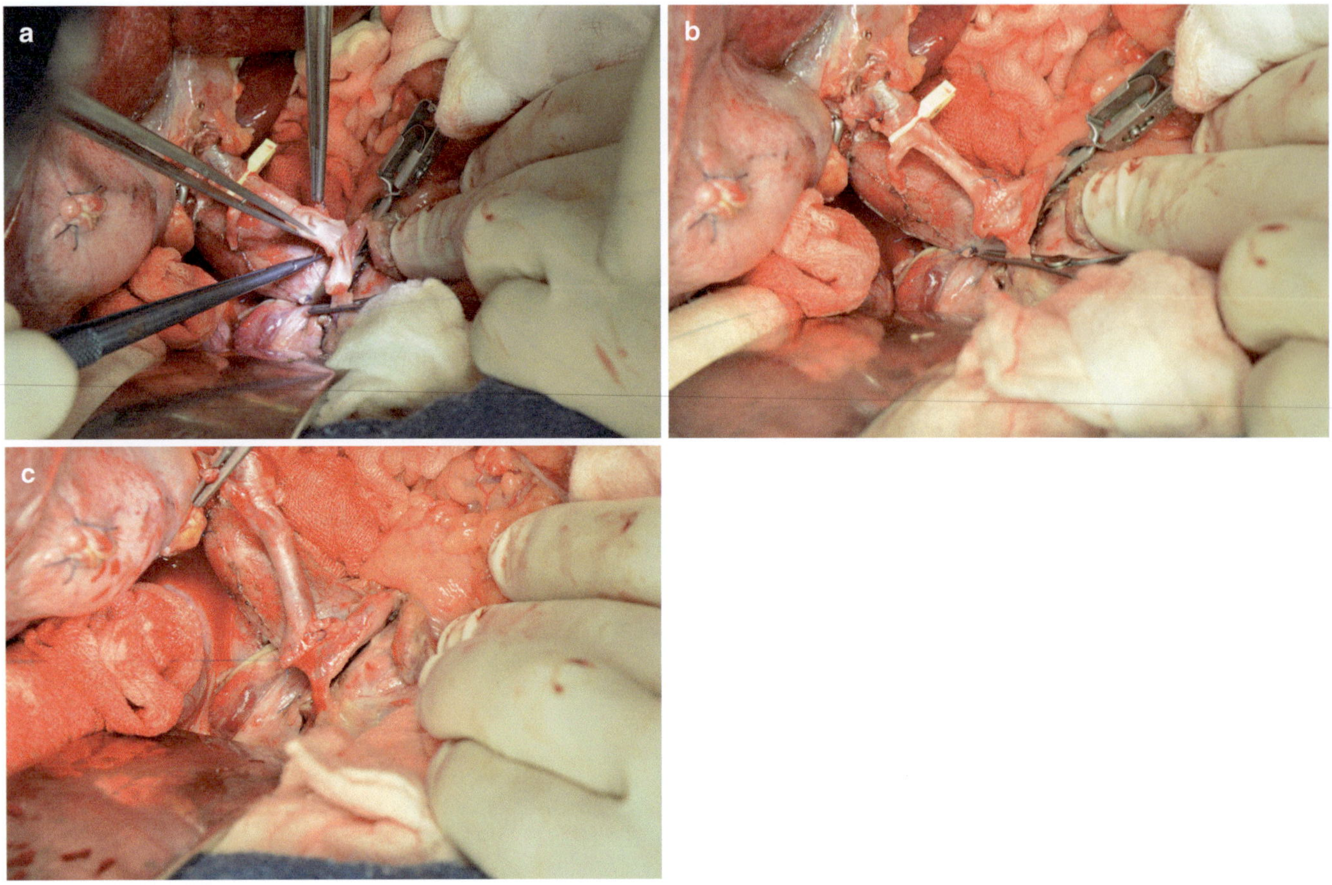

Fig. 7.1 Standard arterial reconstruction (**a**–**c**): anastomosis between the graft common hepatic artery and the junction of the gastroduodenal artery and common hepatic artery

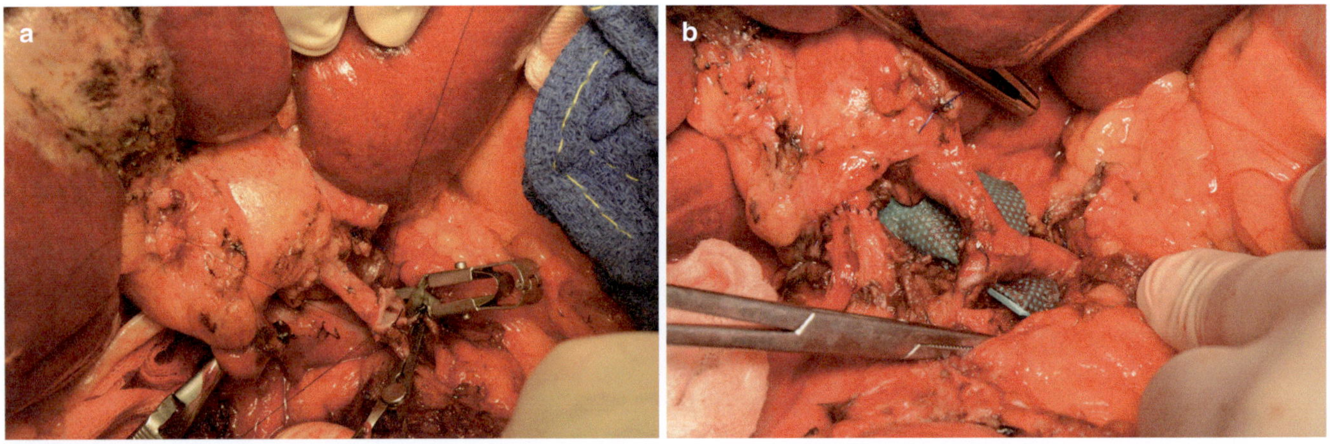

Fig. 7.2 Standard arterial reconstruction (**a**, **b**): anastomosis between the graft common hepatic artery and the junction of the gastroduodenal artery and common hepatic artery

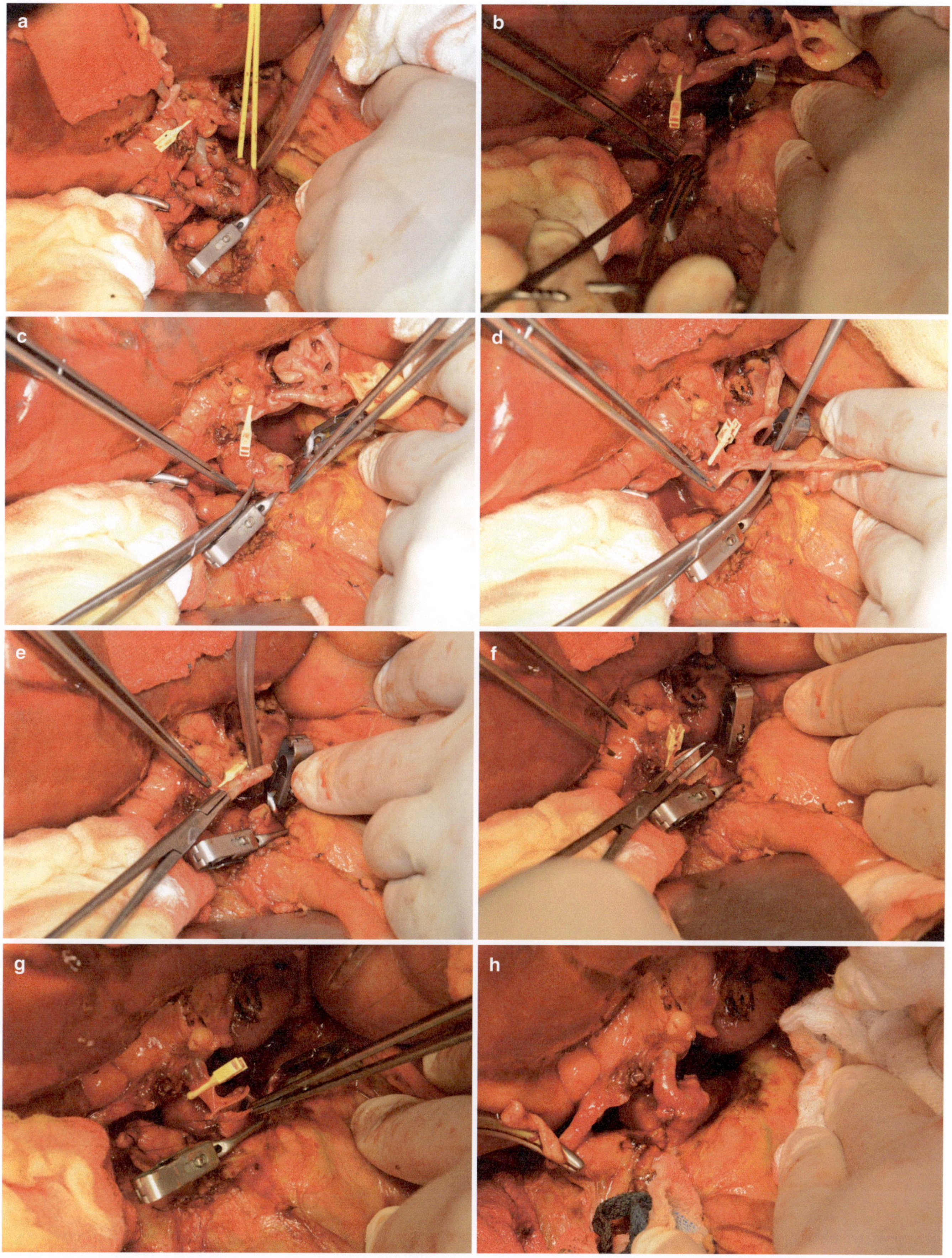

Fig. 7.3 Standard arterial reconstruction (**a–h**): anastomosis between the graft common hepatic artery and the junction of the gastroduodenal artery and common hepatic artery

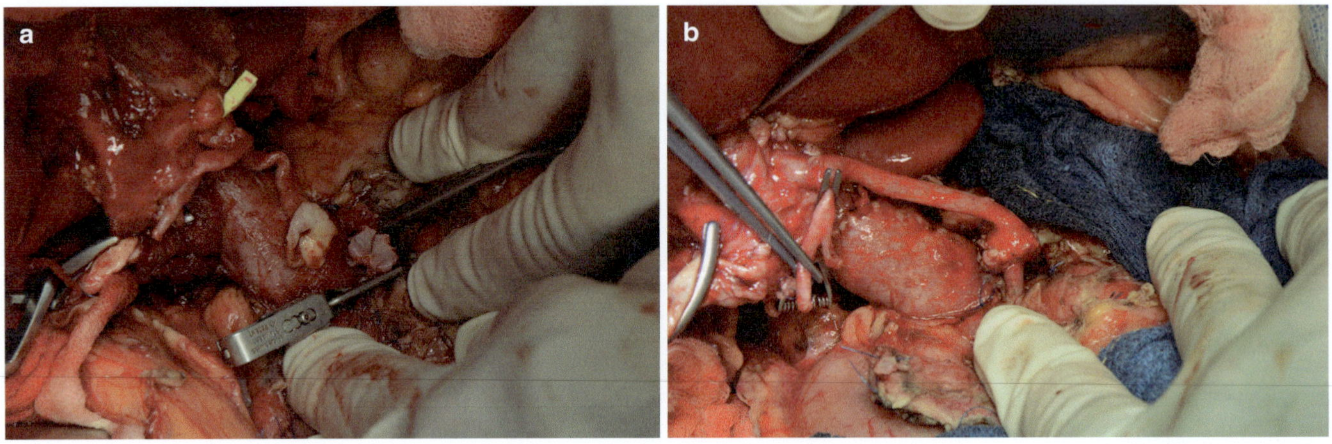

Fig. 7.4 Standard arterial reconstruction (**a**, **b**): anastomosis between the graft common hepatic artery and the junction of the gastroduodenal artery and common hepatic artery

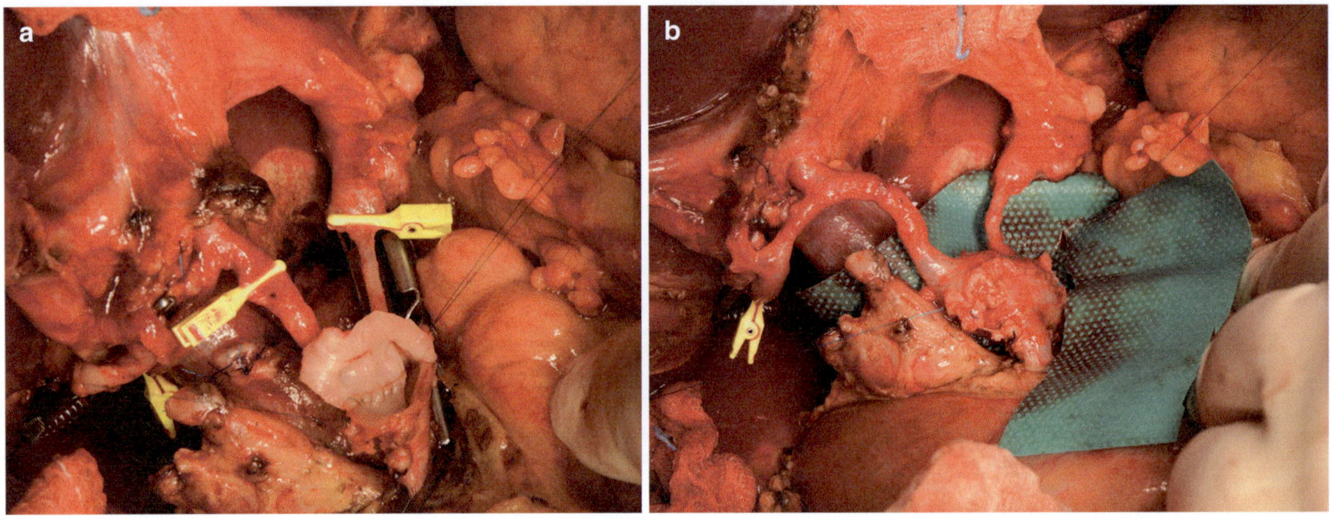

Fig. 7.5 Liver graft with two hepatic arteries (**a**, **b**): anastomosis between the graft celiac trunk (accessory left hepatic artery and common hepatic artery) and the junction of the gastroduodenal artery and common hepatic artery

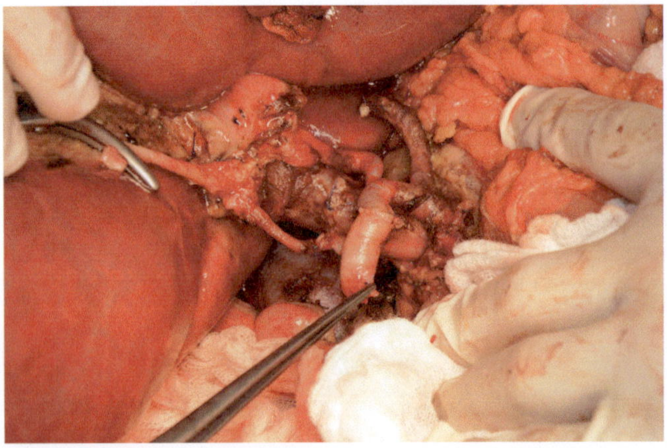

Fig. 7.6 Liver graft with three hepatic arteries: two anastomoses including one between the graft celiac trunk and the junction of the gastroduodenal artery and common hepatic artery and one between the graft splenic artery and the graft superior mesenteric artery

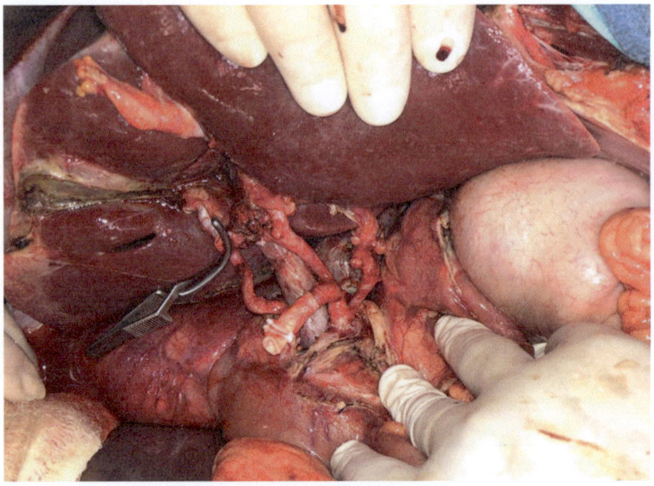

Fig. 7.7 Liver graft with three hepatic arteries: two anastomoses including one between the graft celiac trunk and the junction of the gastroduodenal artery and common hepatic artery and one between the graft splenic artery and the graft superior mesenteric artery

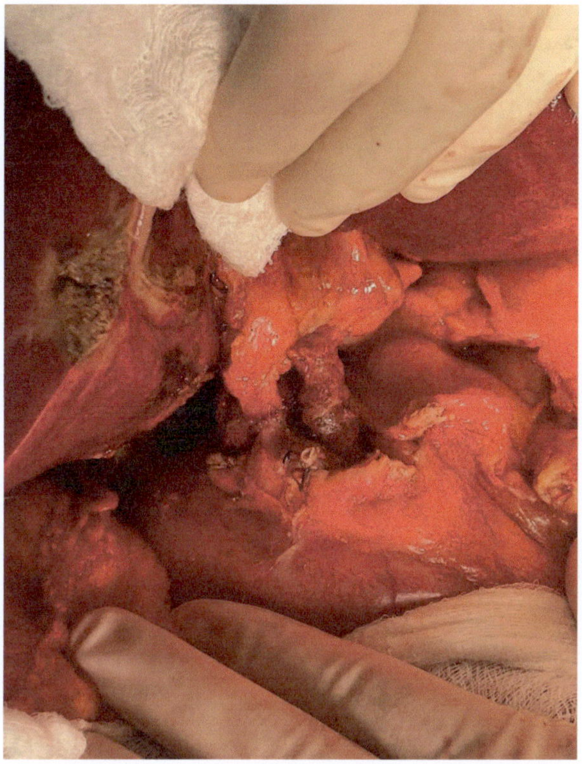

Fig. 7.8 Standard arterial and biliary reconstructions

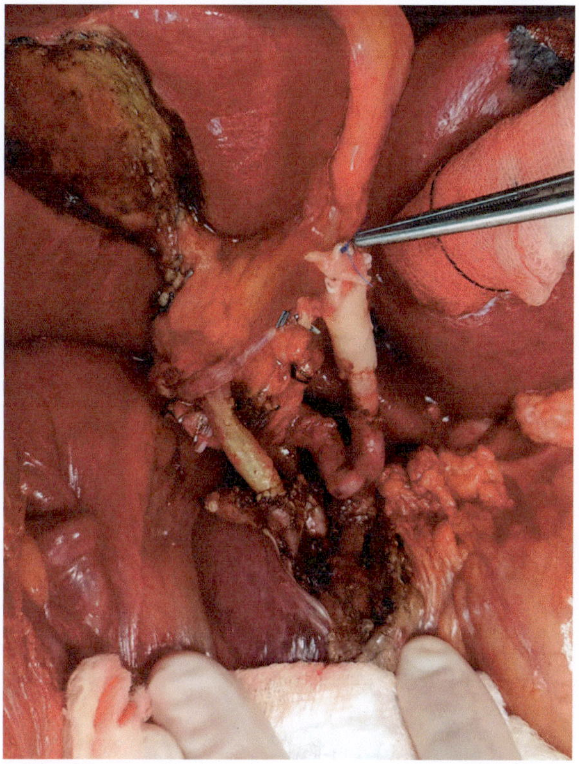

Fig. 7.9 Bilio-biliary anastomosis and arterial reconstructions (graft with two hepatic arteries) with two anastomoses including one between the graft celiac trunk and the junction of the gastroduodenal artery and common hepatic artery and one between the graft splenic artery and the graft superior mesenteric artery

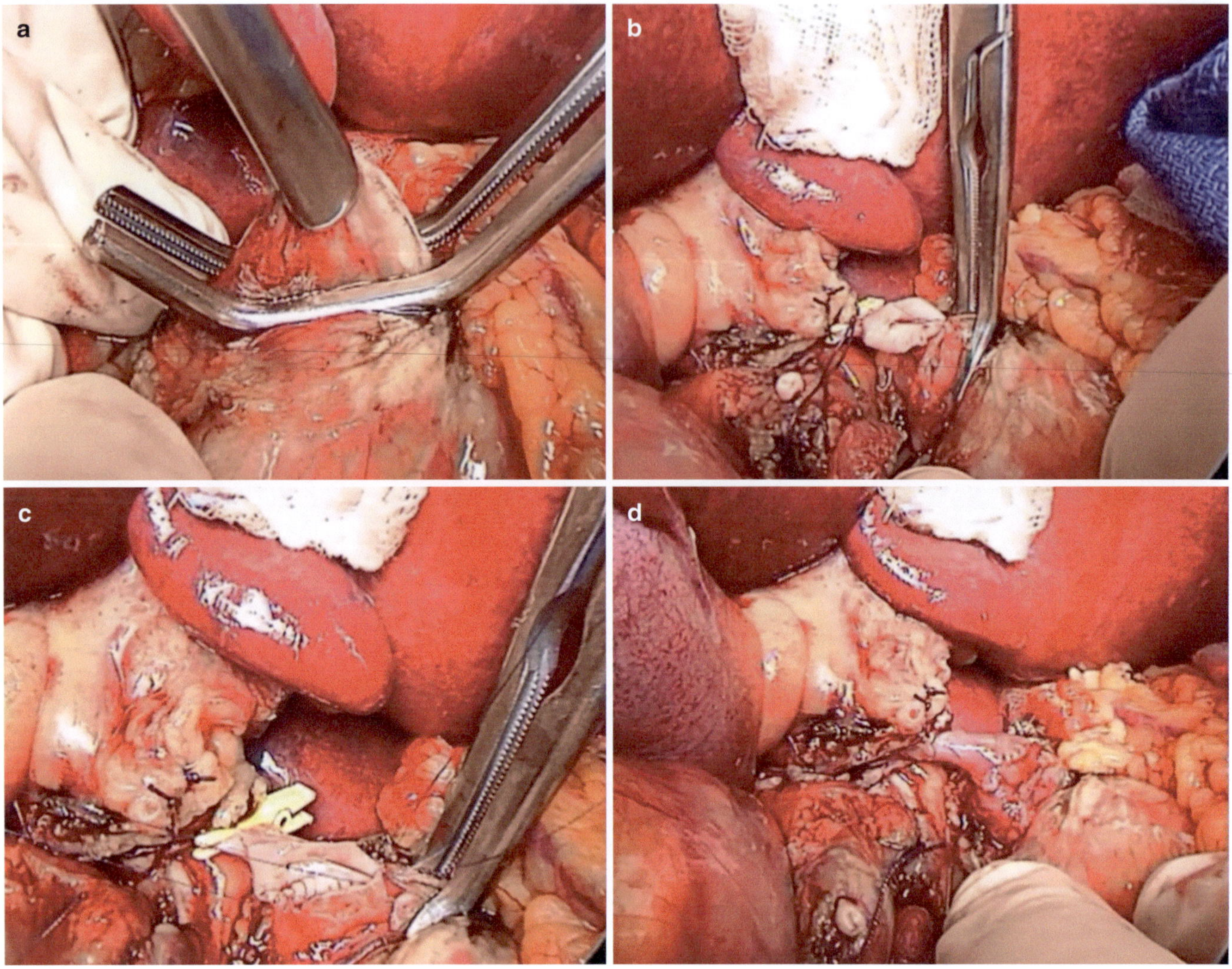

Fig. 7.10 Non-standard arterial reconstruction with an end-to-side arterial anastomosis between the graft hepatic artery and the native splenic artery (**a**–**d**). (**a**) Lateral clamping of the splenic artery. (**b**–**d**) End-to-side anastomosis between the graft common hepatic artery and the splenic artery

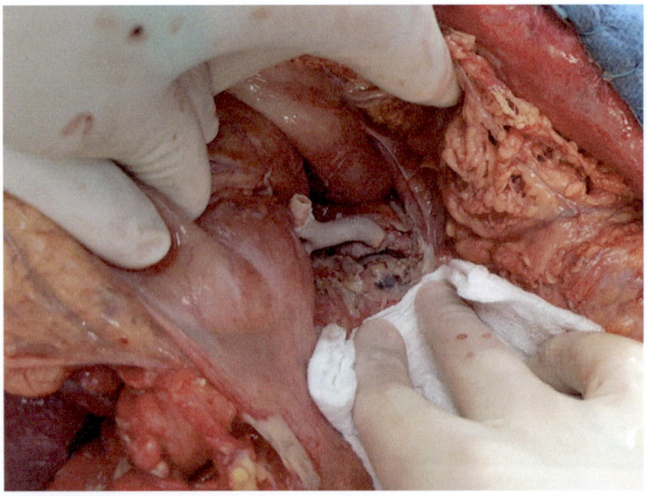

Fig. 7.11 Non-standard arterial reconstruction with an end-to-side arterial anastomosis between the graft hepatic artery and the native splenic artery

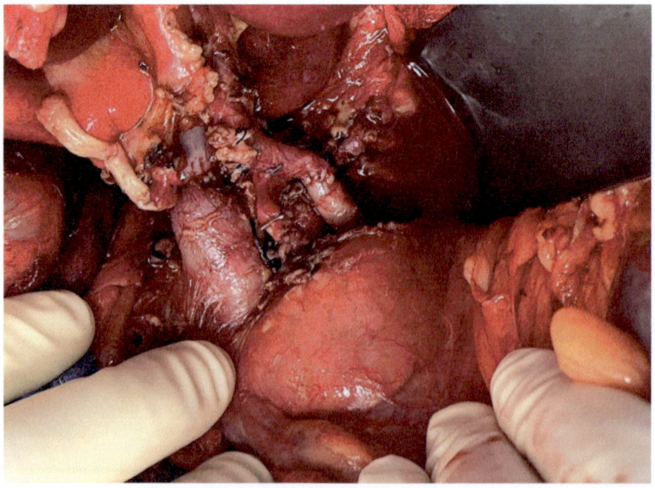

Fig. 7.12 Non-standard arterial reconstruction with an end-to-end arterial anastomosis between the graft hepatic artery and the native splenic artery

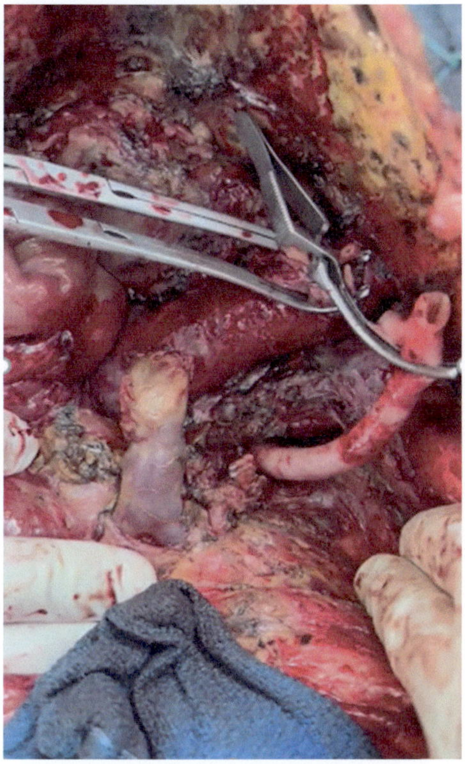

Fig. 7.13 Non-standard arterial reconstruction with anastomosis between the supraceliac aorta and an arterial allograft

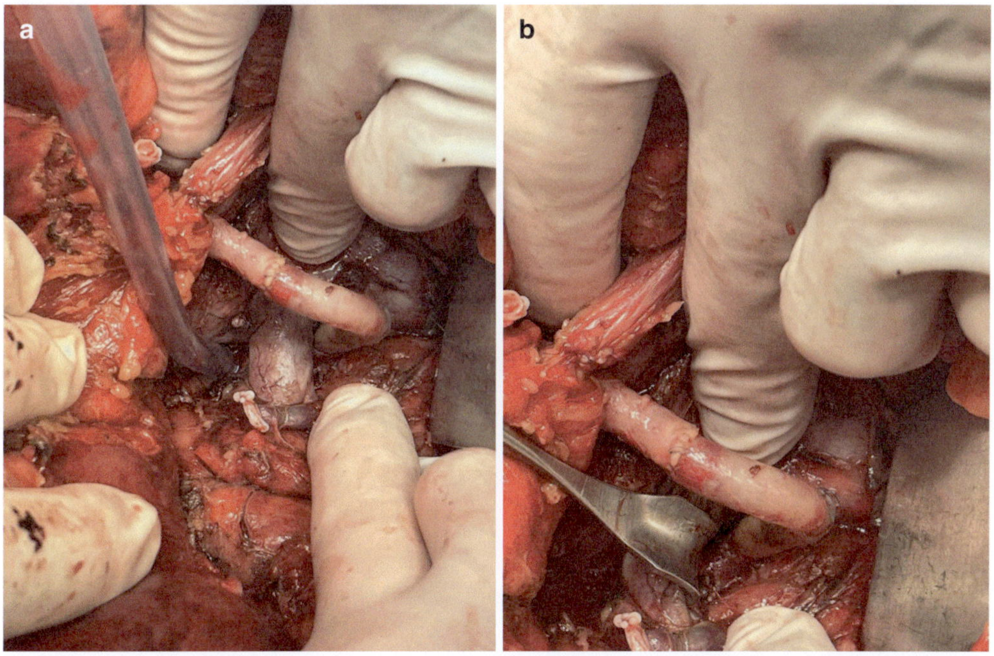

Fig. 7.14 Non-standard arterial reconstruction with an end-to-side anastomosis between the graft hepatic artery and the native right renal artery using an interposed arterial allograft (**a**, **b**)

Reference

1. Yilmaz S, Kutluturk K, Usta S, Akbulut S. Techniques of hepatic arterial reconstruction in liver transplantation. Langenbeck's Arch Surg. 2022;407(7):2607–18. https://doi.org/10.1007/s00423-022-02659-6. Epub 2022 Aug 26.

Back-Table Preparation of a Right Ex Situ Split Graft for Liver Transplantation

8

In France, deceased donor and graft allocation is performed with priority for pediatric recipients. Donor selection for split-liver transplantation is done by pediatric surgeons with a national prioritization of the left graft for a pediatric recipient. The right graft is allocated to an adult. The split procedure is usually performed ex situ using grafts from donation after brain death by either the adult or pediatric team [1].

C. Lim et al., *Atlas of Liver Transplantation*, https://doi.org/10.1007/978-3-031-85264-0_8

Full Right Graft (G15678) (Figs. 8.1, 8.2, 8.3, 8.4, 8.5, 8.6, 8.7, 8.8, 8.9, 8.10, 8.11, 8.12, 8.13, 8.14, 8.15, 8.16, 8.17, 8.18, 8.19, 8.20, 8.21, and 8.22)

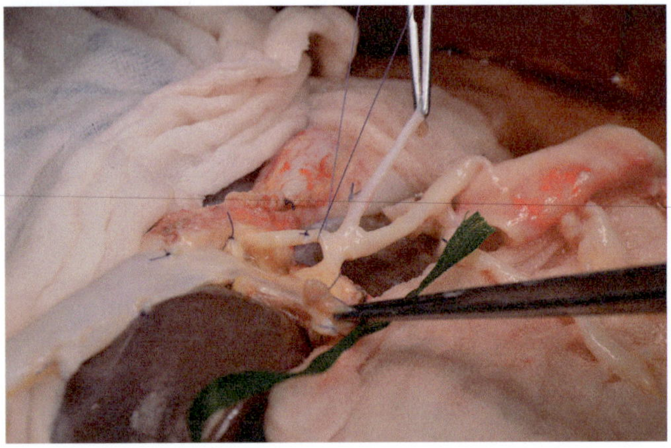

Fig. 8.1 Dissection of the right branch of the hepatic artery

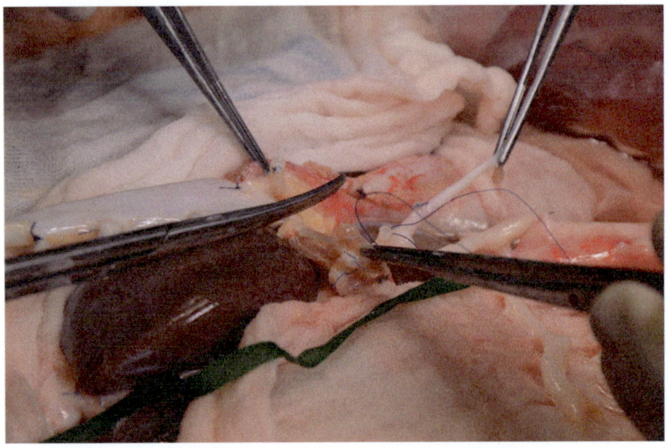

Fig. 8.2 Division of the right branch of the hepatic artery

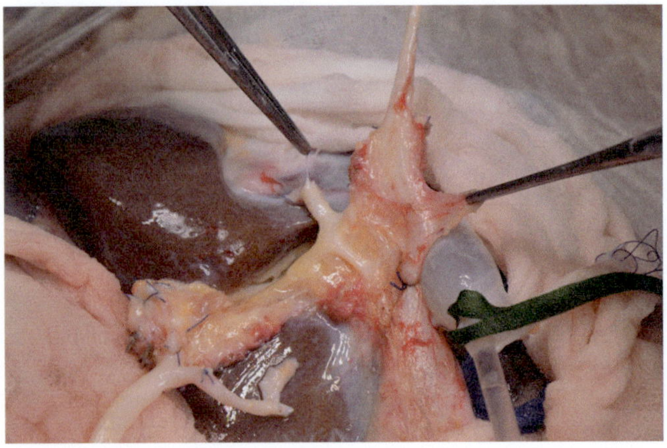

Fig. 8.3 Right branch of the hepatic artery

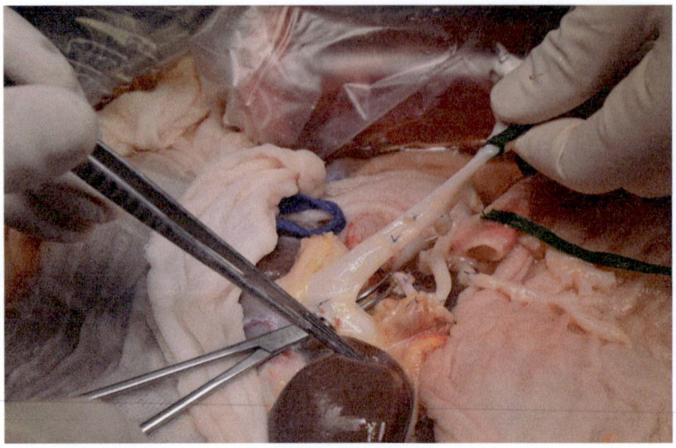

Fig. 8.4 Dissection of the left portal branch

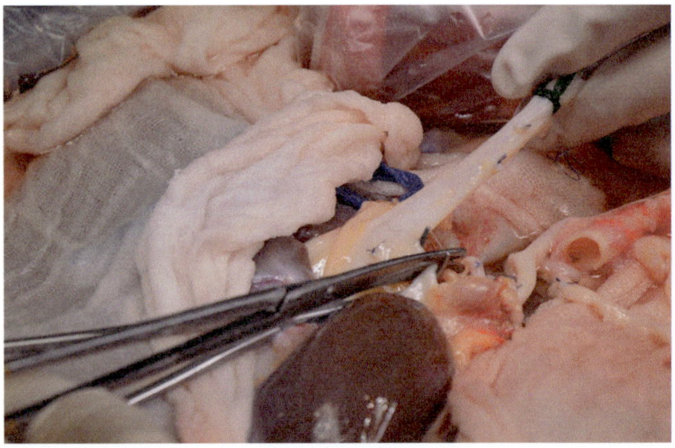

Fig. 8.5 Division of the left portal branch

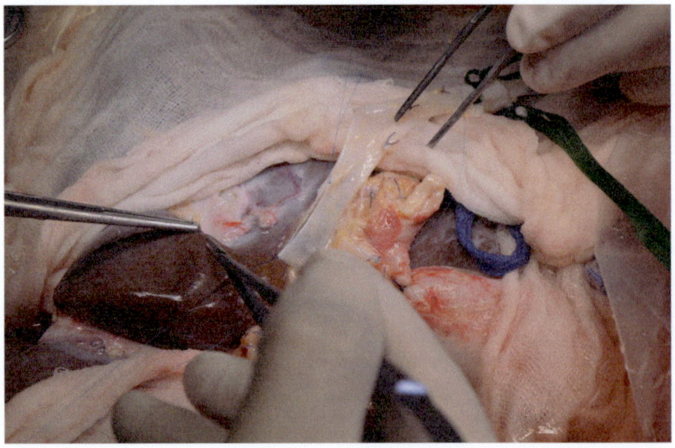

Fig. 8.6 Closure of the hole of the left portal branch

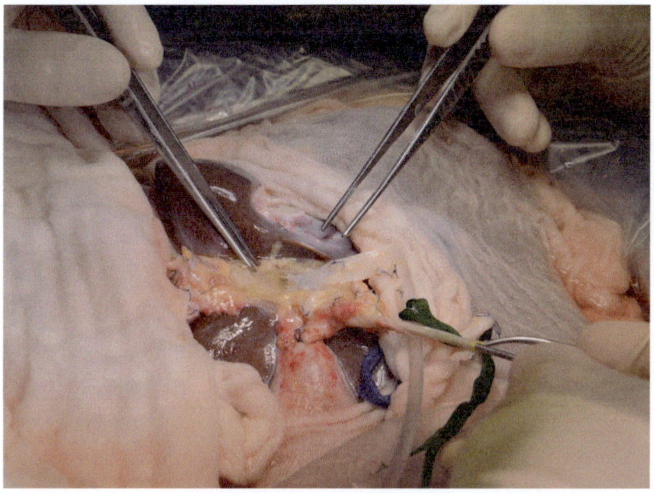

Fig. 8.7 The portal trunk for the extended right graft (G145678)

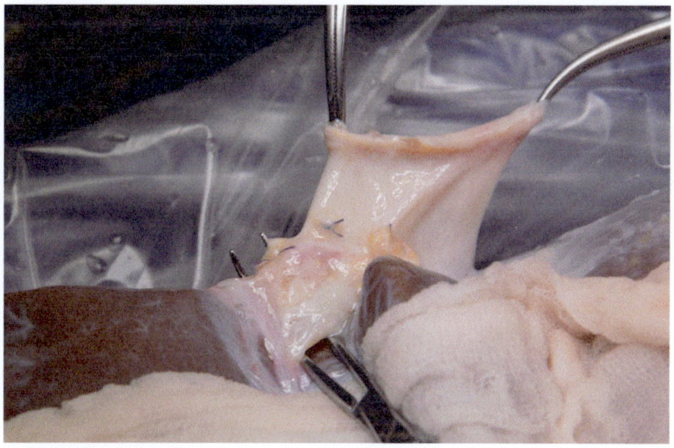

Fig. 8.10 Dissection of the left hepatic vein

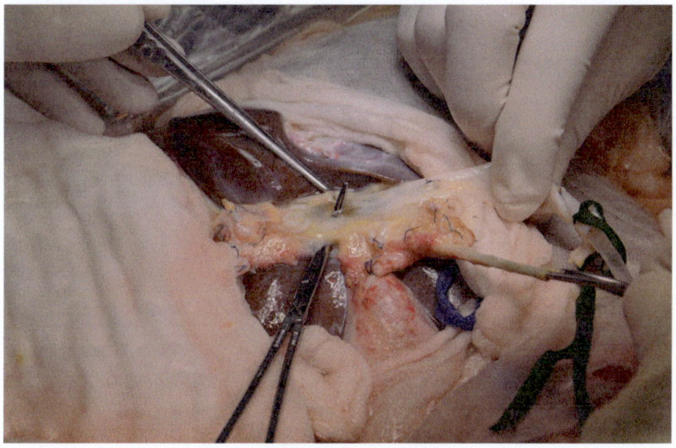

Fig. 8.8 Dissection of the left bile duct

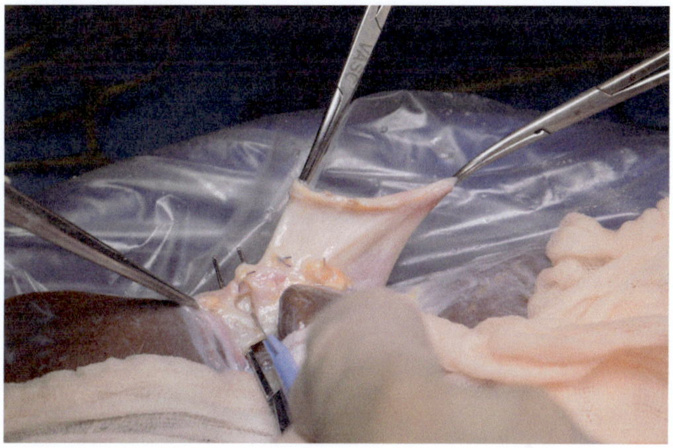

Fig. 8.11 Division of the left hepatic vein

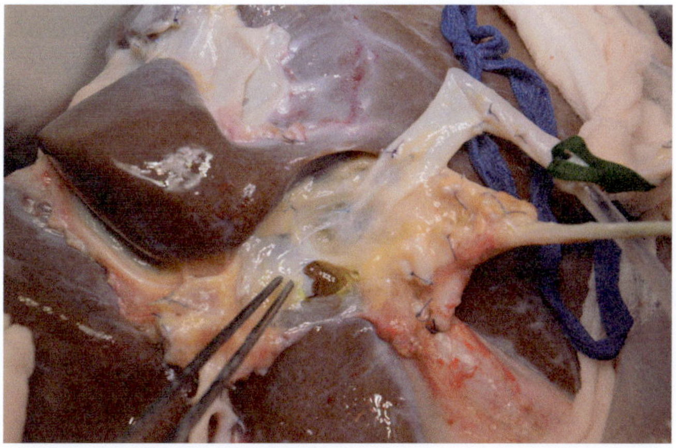

Fig. 8.9 Division of the left bile duct

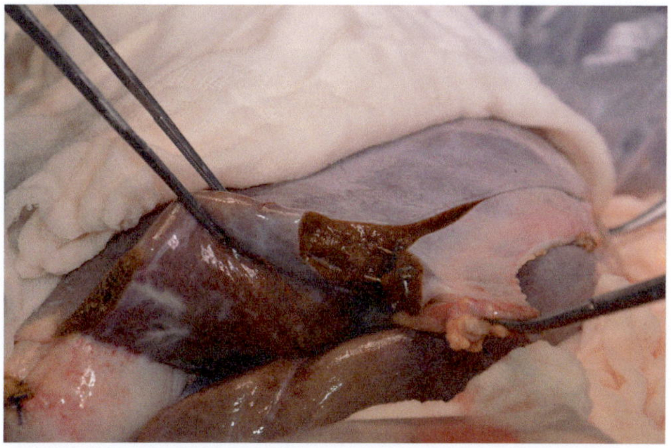

Fig. 8.12 Liver transection to obtain the extended right graft (G145678)

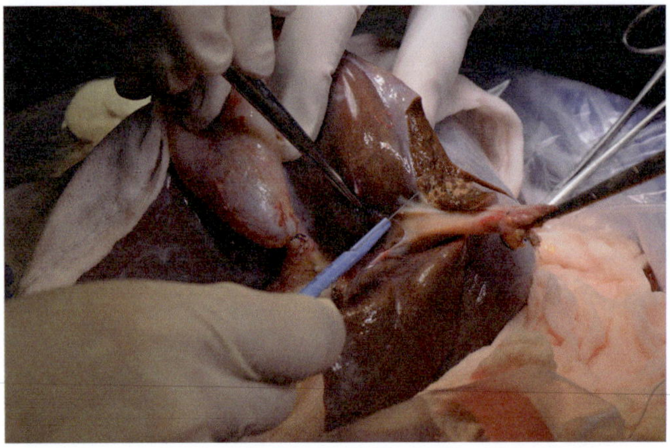

Fig. 8.13 Dissection of the portal branch of segment IV

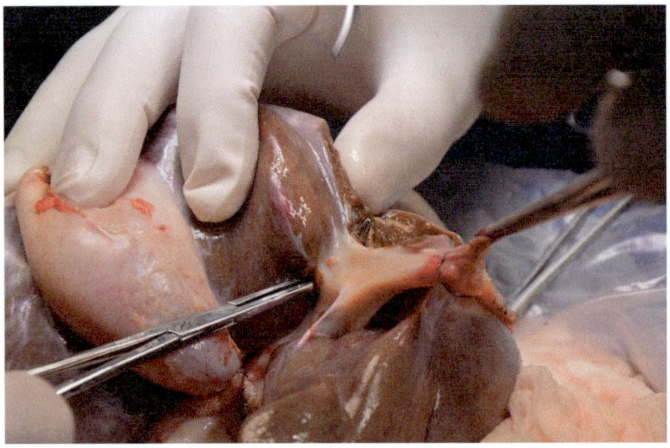

Fig. 8.14 Dissection of the portal branch of segment IV

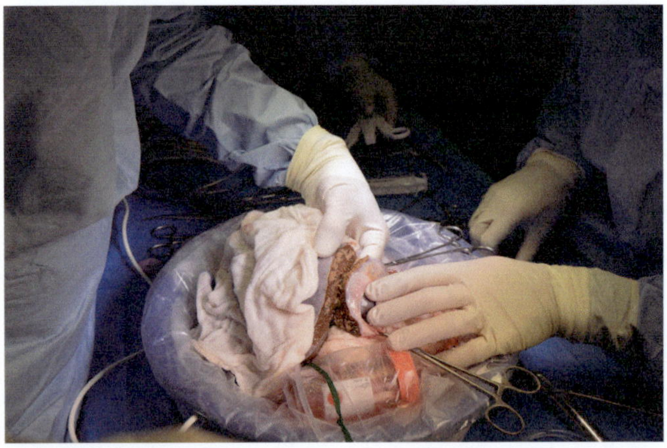

Fig. 8.15 Liver transection

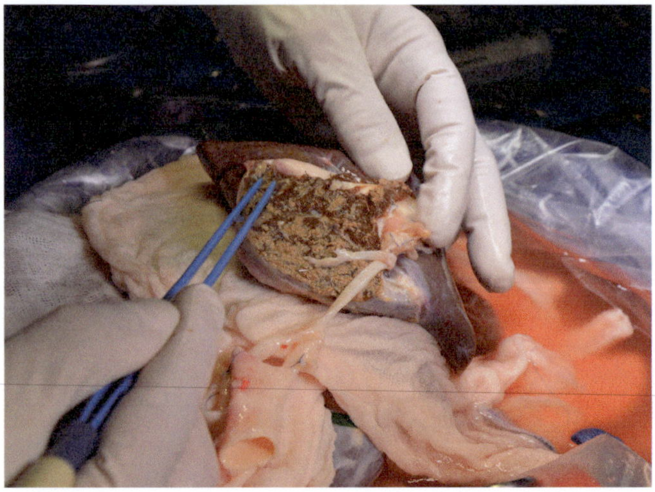

Fig. 8.16 Left graft (G23) including the entire arterial axis

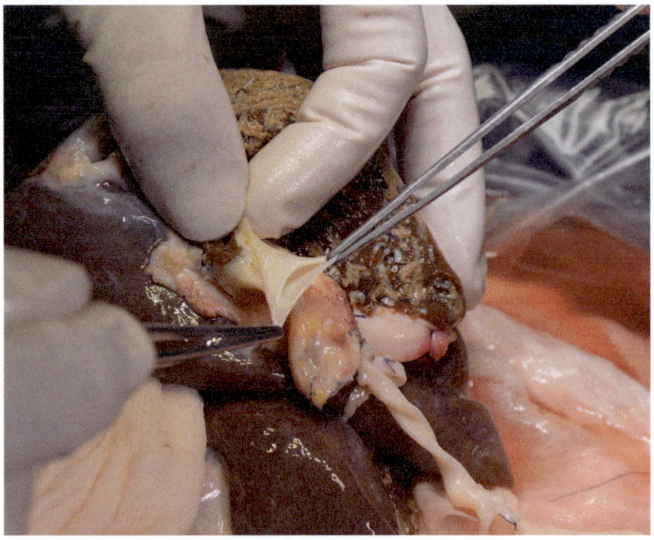

Fig. 8.17 Left portal vein of G23

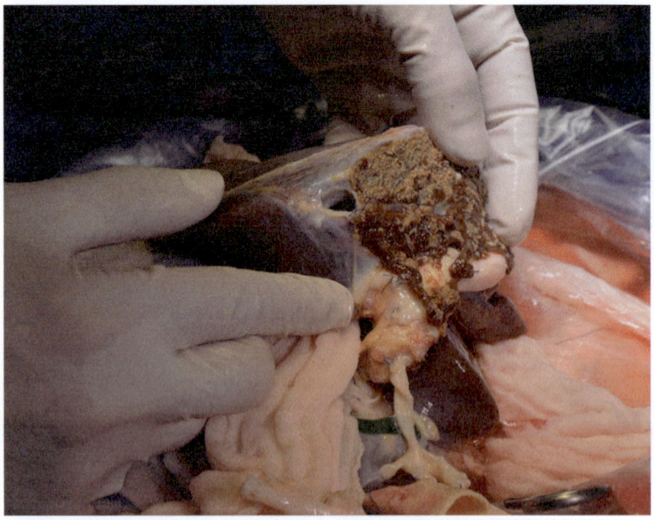

Fig. 8.18 Left hepatic vein of G23

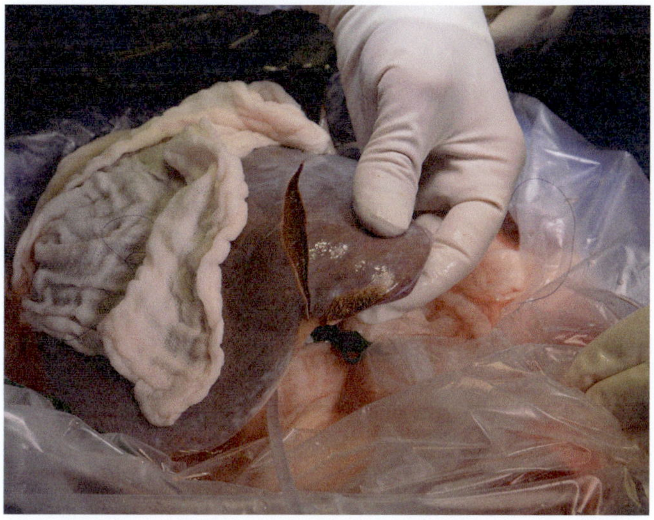

Fig. 8.19 Segmentectomy IV of the extended right graft (G45678)

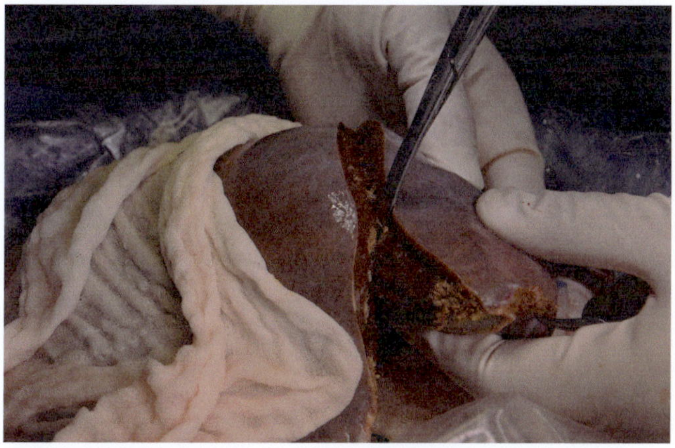

Fig. 8.20 Segmentectomy IV of the extended right graft (G45678)

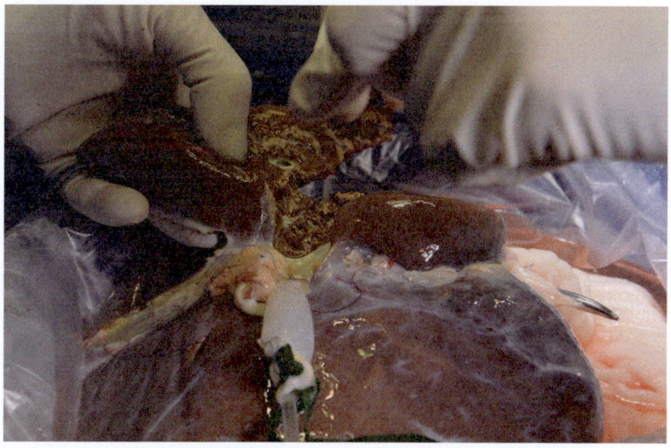

Fig. 8.21 Segmentectomy IV of the extended right graft (G45678)

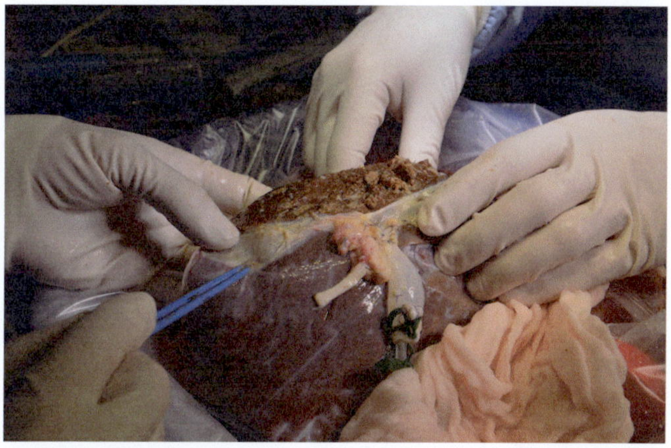

Fig. 8.22 Cholecystectomy

Full Right Graft (G15678)—Middle Hepatic Vein (MHV) (Figs. 8.23, 8.24, 8.25, 8.26, 8.27, and 8.28)

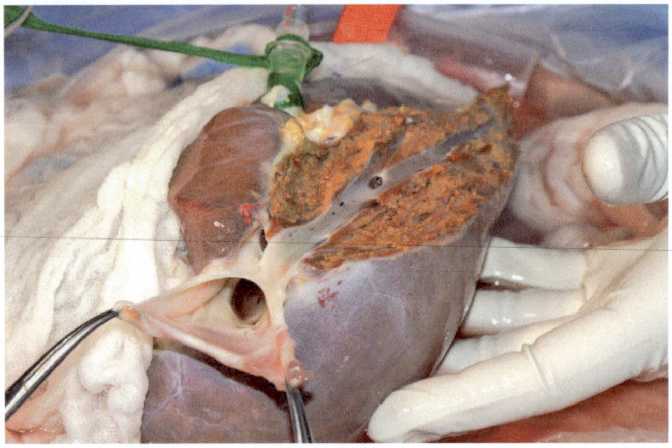

Fig. 8.23 Full right graft with MHV (G15678—MHV)

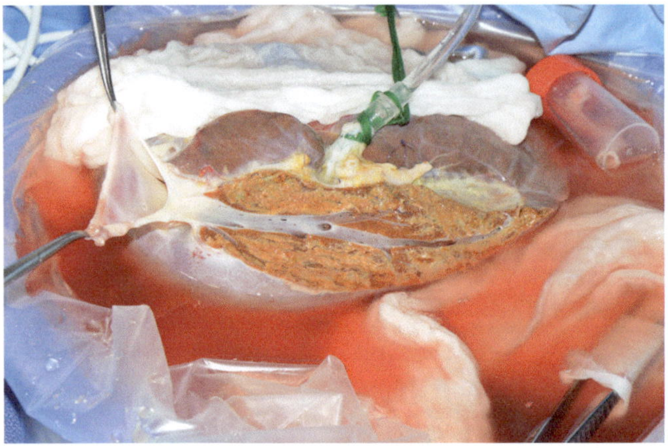

Fig. 8.24 Full right graft with MHV (G15678—MHV)

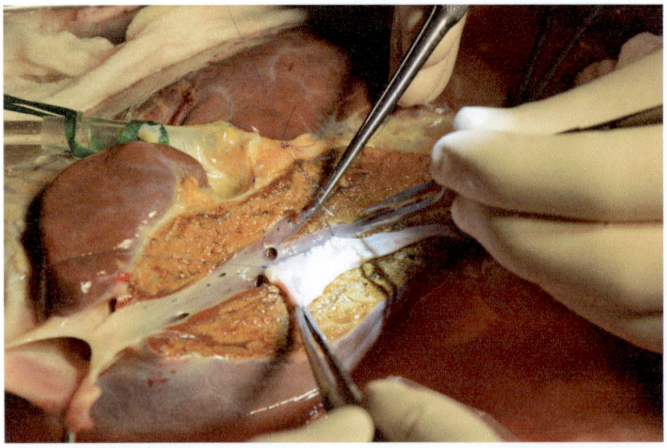

Fig. 8.25 Reconstruction of the middle hepatic vein using a femoral venous allograft

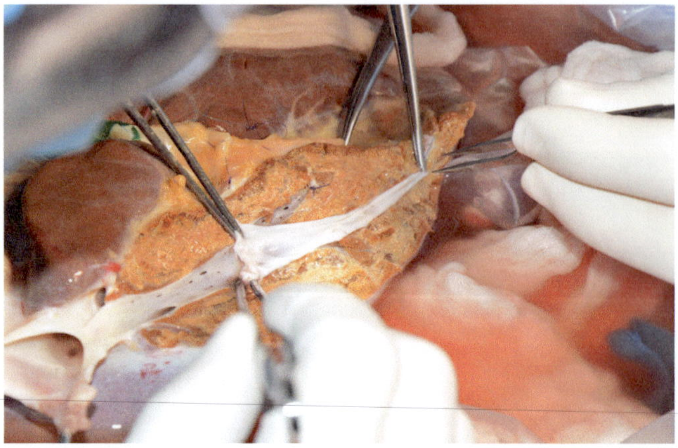

Fig. 8.26 Reconstruction of the middle hepatic vein using a femoral venous allograft

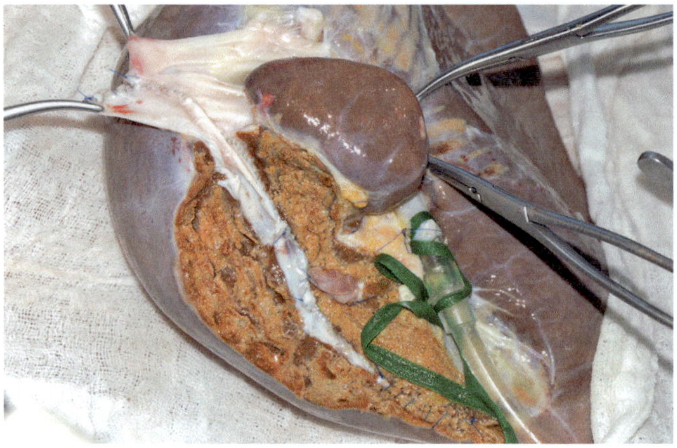

Fig. 8.27 G15678 with the reconstructed middle hepatic vein

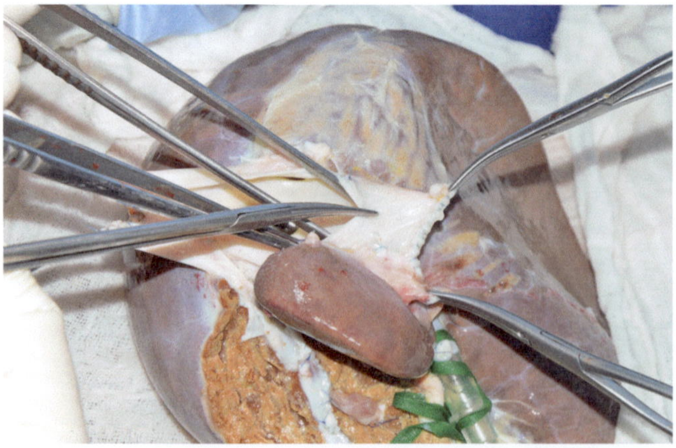

Fig. 8.28 Incision of the posterior wall of the inferior vena cava

Full Right Graft (G5678) (Figs. 8.29 and 8.30)

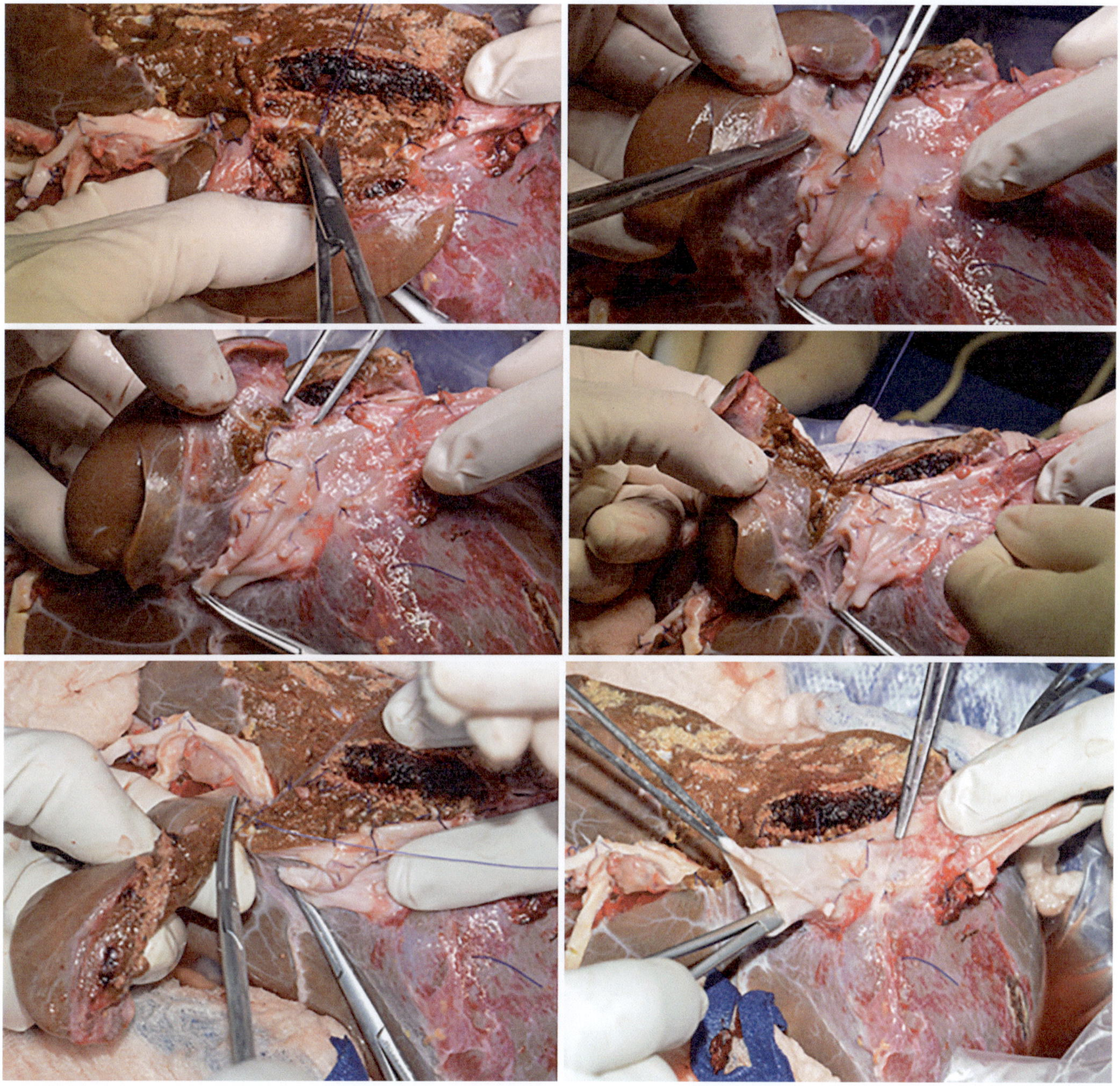

Fig. 8.29 Segmentectomy I of the G15678

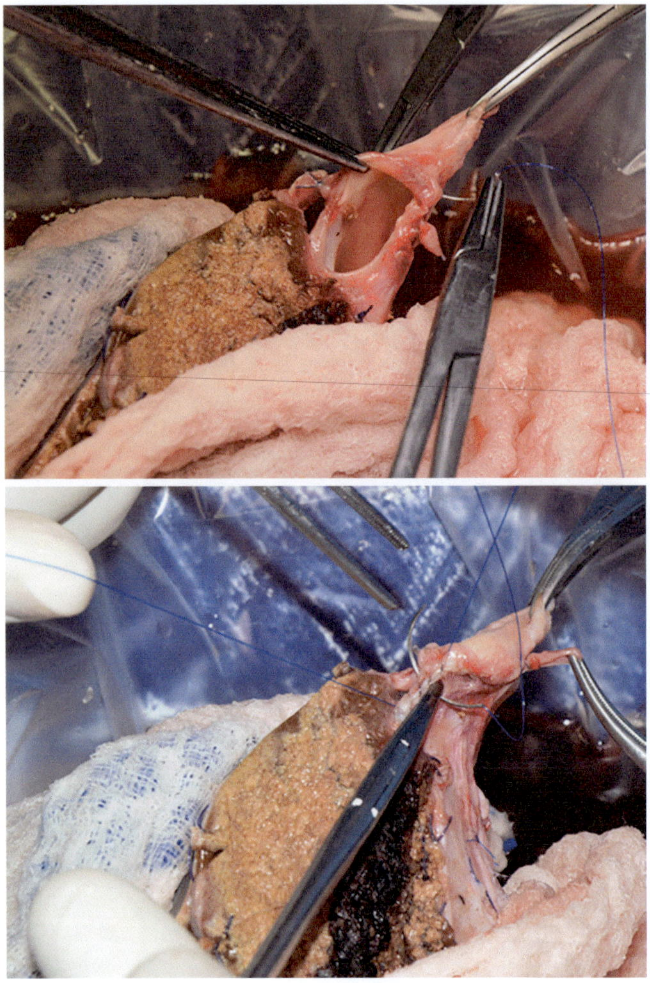

Fig. 8.30 Closure of the hole of the left hepatic vein

Extended Right (G145678) and Left (G23) Grafts (Figs. 8.31, 8.32, 8.33, 8.34, and 8.35)

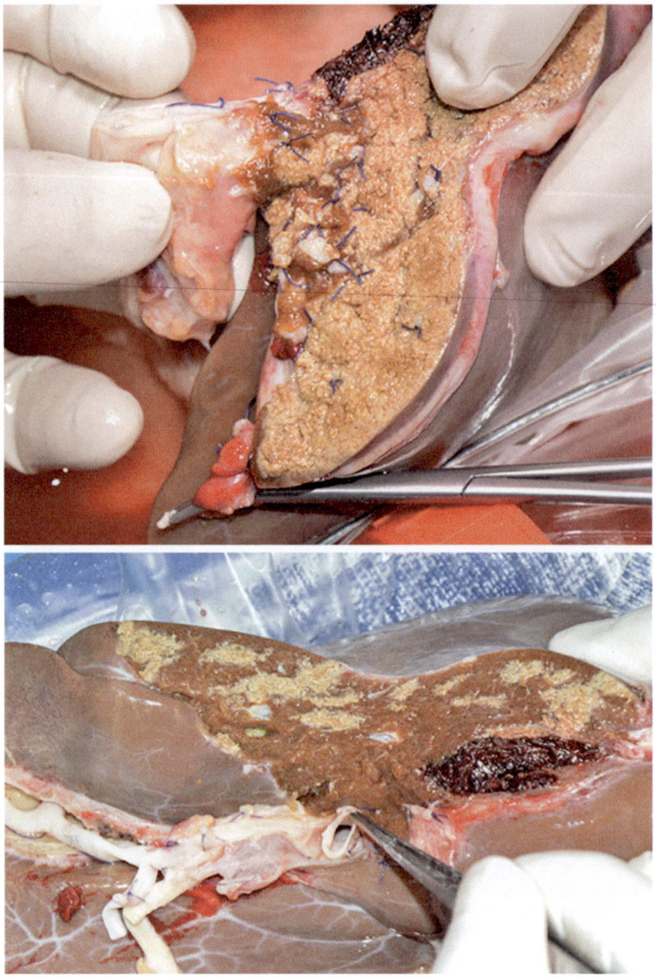

Fig. 8.31 G23 (entire arterial axis, left bile duct and portal vein) and G145678 (common bile duct, right branch of the portal vein and right branch of the hepatic artery)

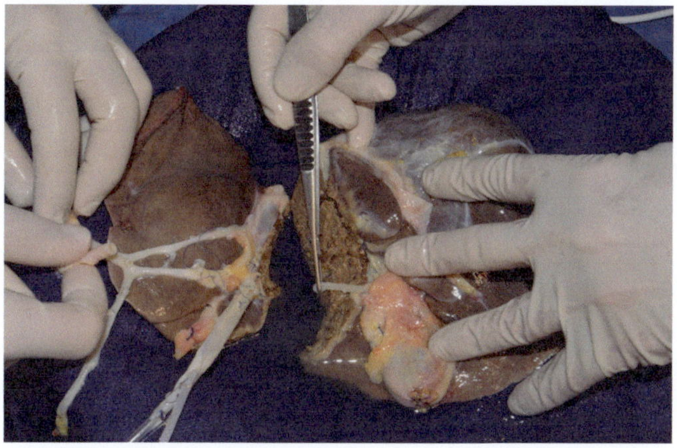

Fig. 8.32 G23 (entire arterial axis, left bile duct and portal vein) and G145678 (common bile duct, right branch of the portal vein and right branch of the hepatic artery)

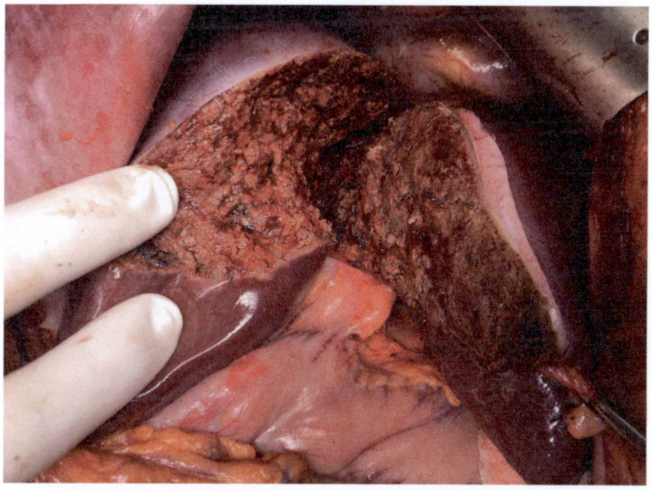

Fig. 8.34 In situ split graft for adult liver transplantation (G123 and G45678)

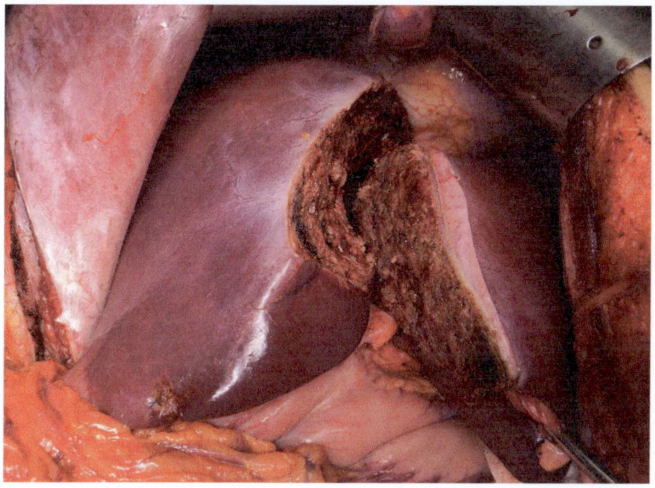

Fig. 8.33 In situ split graft for adult liver transplantation (G123 and G45678)

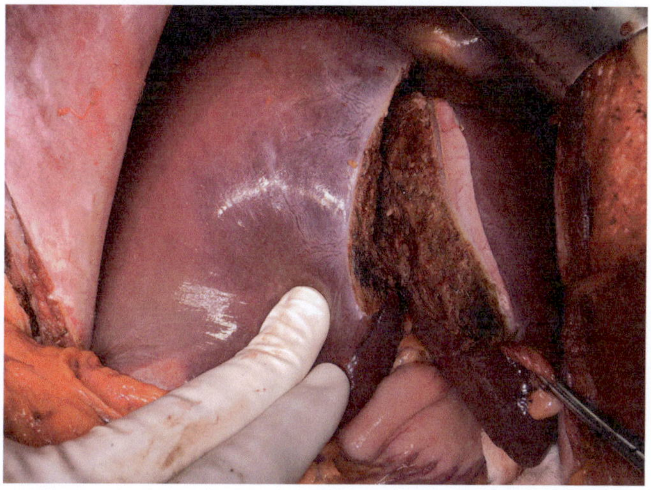

Fig. 8.35 In situ split graft for adult liver transplantation (G123 and G45678)

Reference

1. Boulanger N, Muller X, Dondero F, Golse N, Goumard C, Breton A, et al. Right ex-situ split grafts for adult liver transplantation: a multicenter benchmarking analysis. Ann Surg. 2024; https://doi.org/10.1097/SLA.0000000000006401.

9 Right Split Ex Situ Graft Implantation

During implantation of the right split graft, the continuity of each anastomosis is restored as for a whole graft implantation. As for the arterial anastomotic site, a single arterial branch (right branch of the hepatic artery) is usually present for anastomosis (Figs. 9.1, 9.2, 9.3, 9.4, 9.5, 9.6, 9.7, 9.8, 9.9, 9.10, 9.11, 9.12, 9.13, 9.14, 9.15, 9.16, 9.17, 9.18, 9.19, 9.20, 9.21, 9.22, 9.23, and 9.24) [1, 2].

C. Lim et al., *Atlas of Liver Transplantation*, https://doi.org/10.1007/978-3-031-85264-0_9

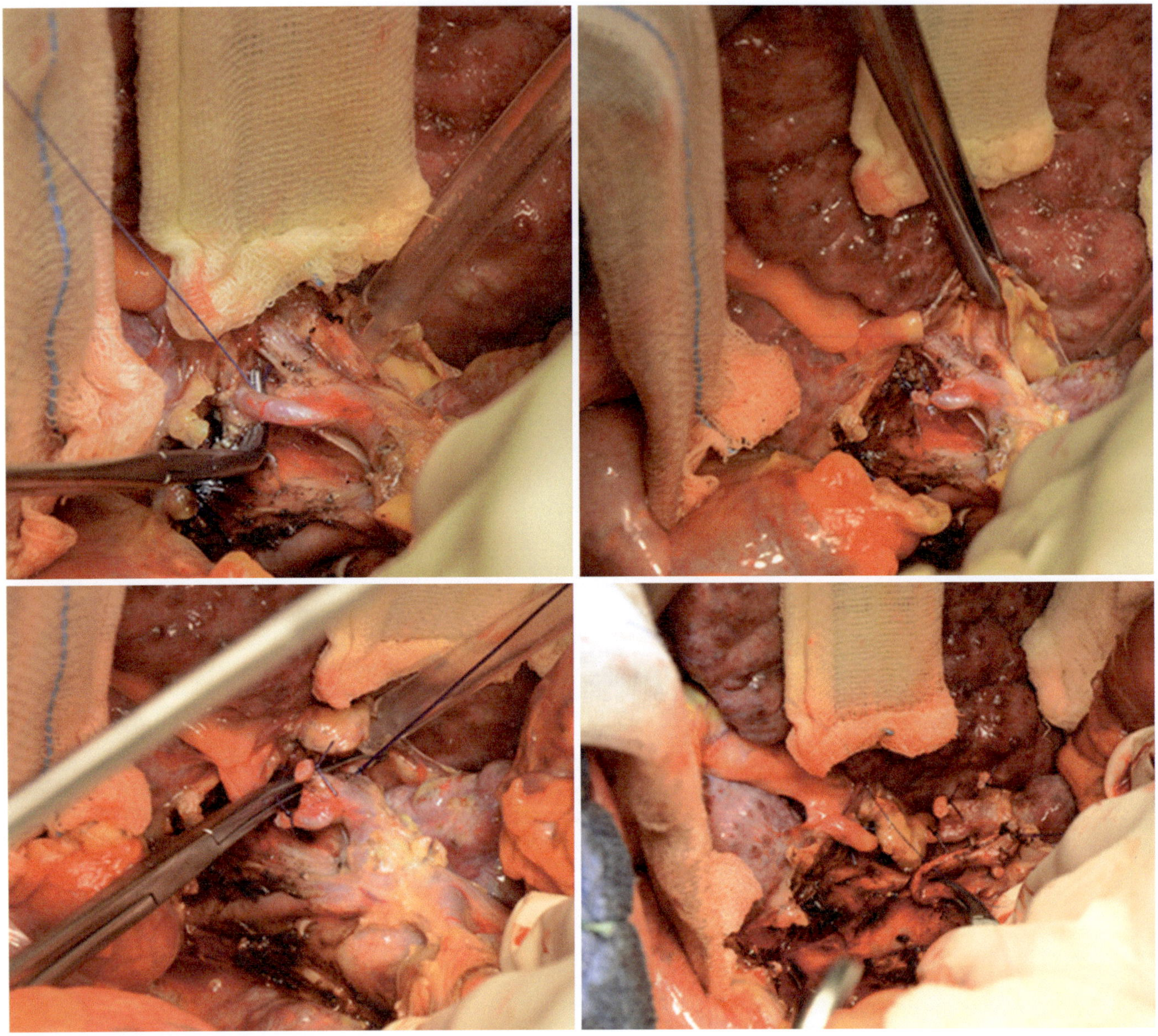

Fig. 9.1 Dissection of the anterior and posterior branches of the right hepatic artery in the adult recipient

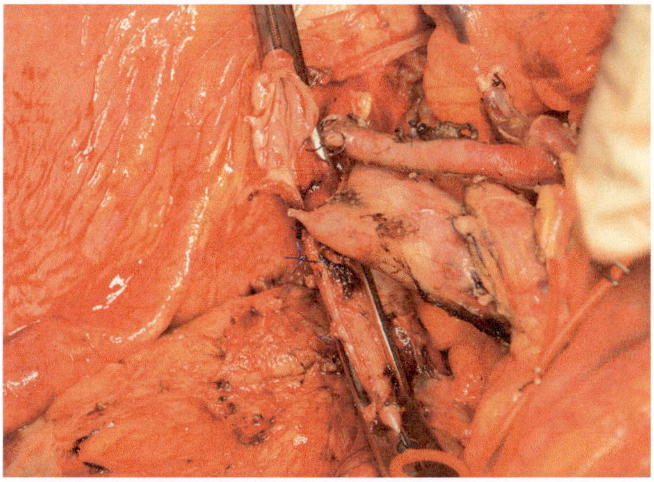

Fig. 9.2 Intraoperative view after total hepatectomy (inferior vena cava clamped using a Satinsky forceps)

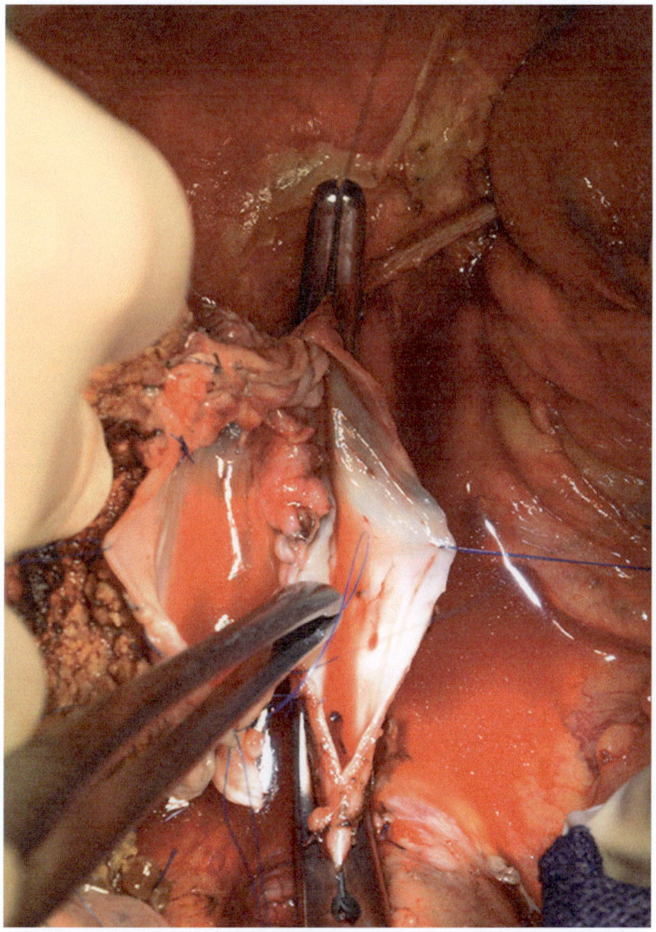

Fig. 9.3 Piggyback caval anastomosis technique: posterior wall

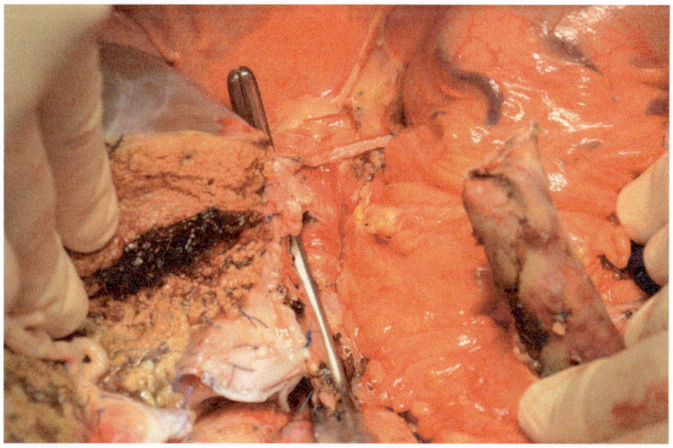

Fig. 9.4 Caval anastomosis before unclamping

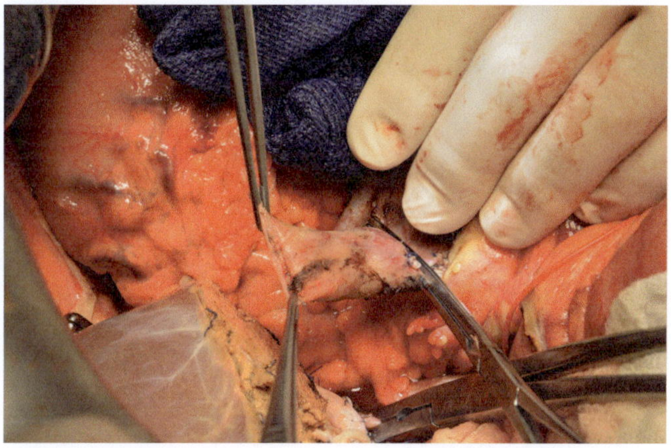

Fig. 9.5 Clamping of the native portal vein before porto-portal anastomosis

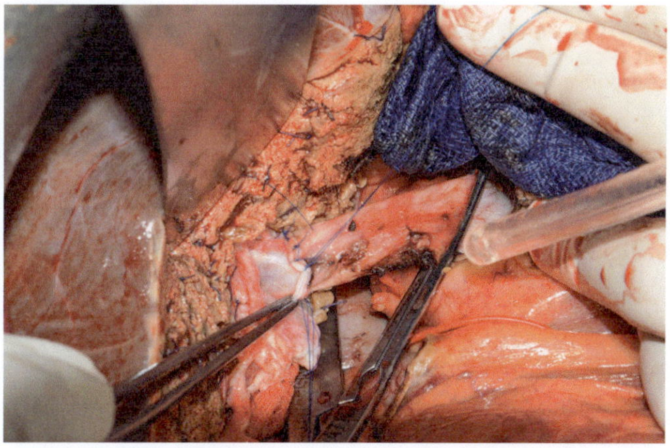

Fig. 9.6 Porto-portal anastomosis

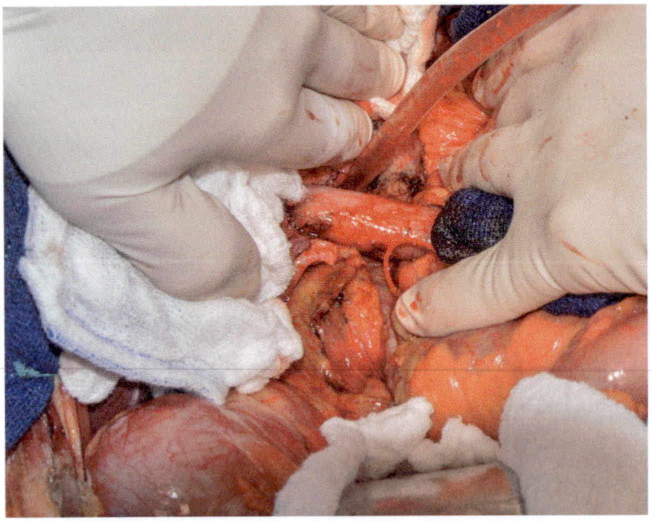

Fig. 9.7 Unclamping of the caval and portal anastomoses and compression of the transection plane of the right split graft

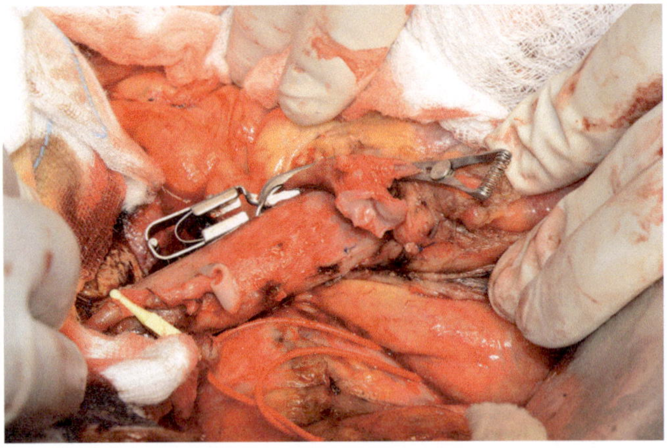

Fig. 9.8 Right split graft with an entire arterial axis including the superior mesenteric artery patch and the accessory right hepatic artery. The anastomosis is performed between the graft superior mesenteric artery patch and the junction of the gastroduodenal artery and the common hepatic artery

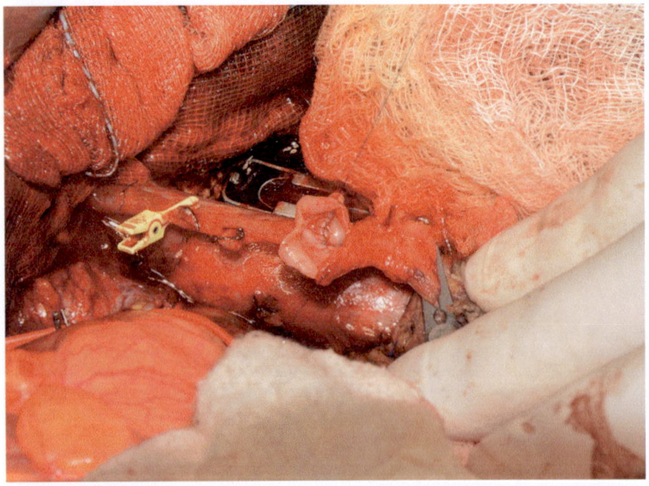

Fig. 9.9 Posterior wall of the arterial anastomosis between the graft superior mesenteric artery patch and the junction of the gastroduodenal artery and the common hepatic artery

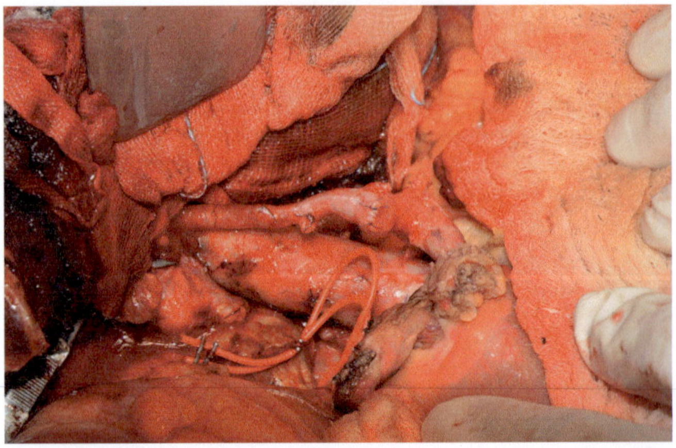

Fig. 9.10 Arterial anastomosis between the graft superior mesenteric artery patch and the junction of the gastroduodenal artery and the common hepatic artery

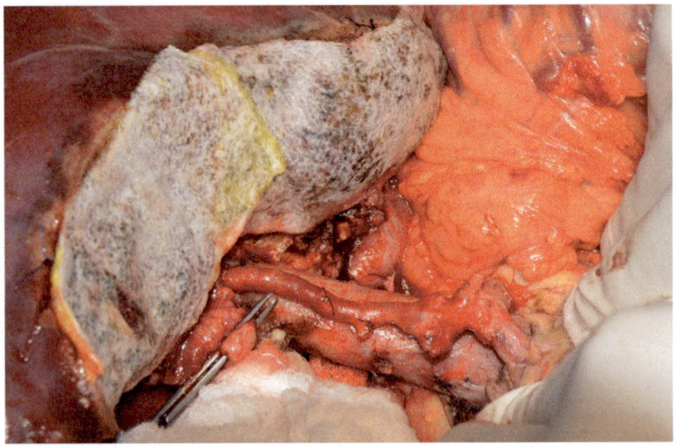

Fig. 9.11 Final aspect of the transection plane of the right spit graft after arterial anastomosis

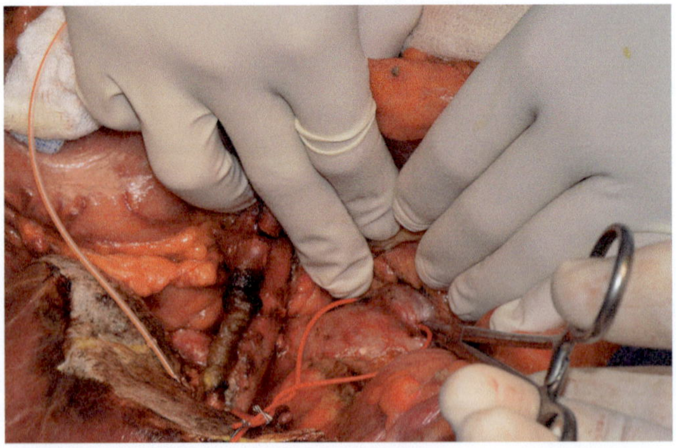

Fig. 9.12 Dissection of the left renal vein

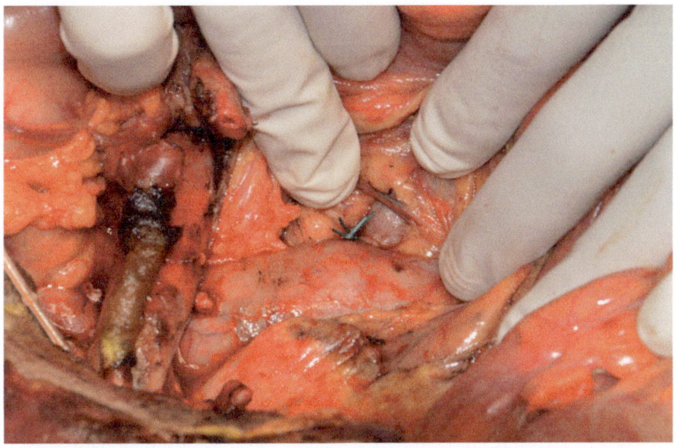

Fig. 9.13 Ligation of the left renal vein to avoid a steal syndrome

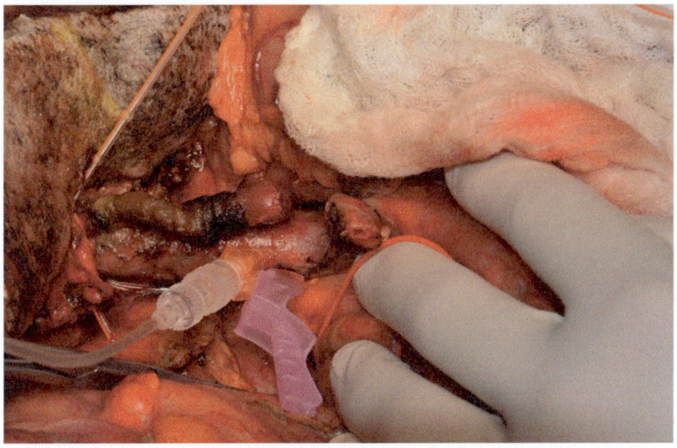

Fig. 9.14 Insertion of an external biliary drain from the left hepatic duct before biliary anastomosis

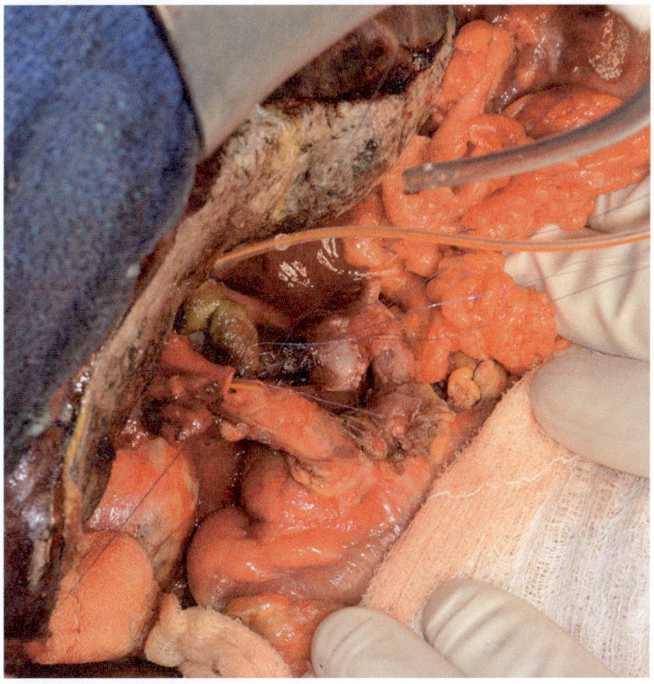

Fig. 9.15 Posterior wall of the bilio-biliary anastomosis

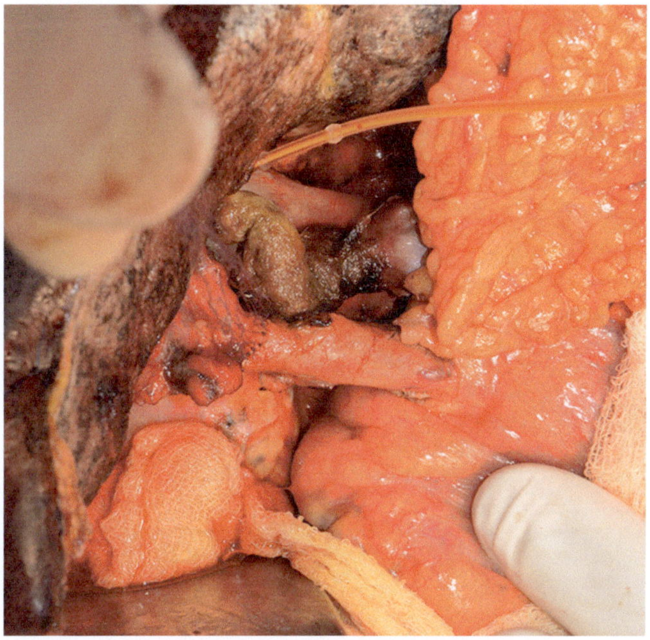

Fig. 9.16 Completion of the bilio-biliary anastomosis with an external biliary drain

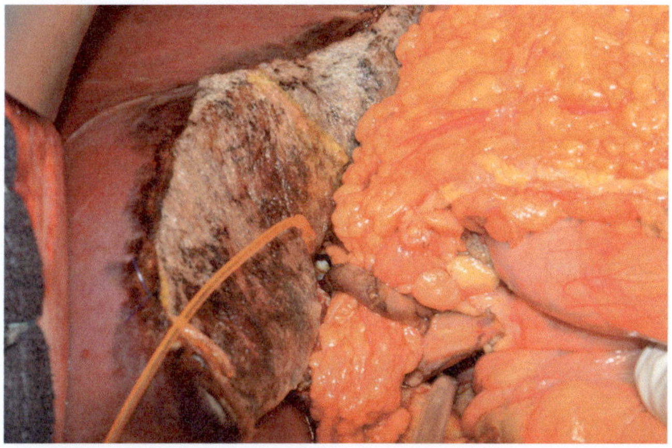

Fig. 9.17 Interposition of omental flap to prevent arterial kinking

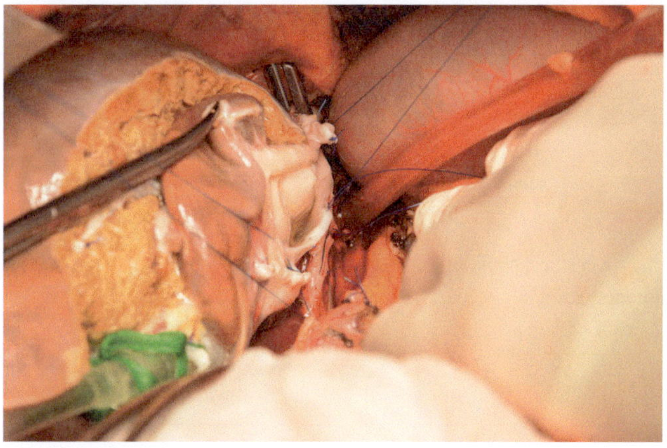

Fig. 9.18 Caval anastomosis of the G15678-MHV

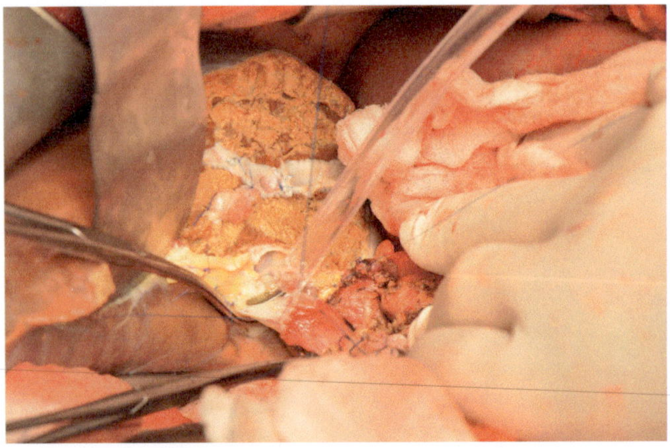

Fig. 9.19 Portal anastomosis of the G15678-MHV

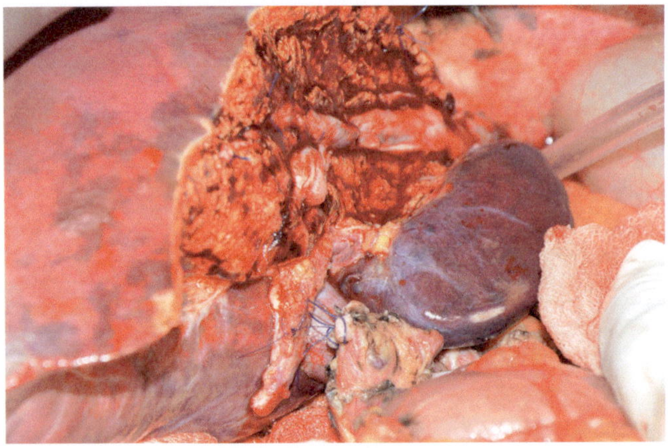

Fig. 9.20 G15678-MHV: the middle hepatic vein has been reconstructed

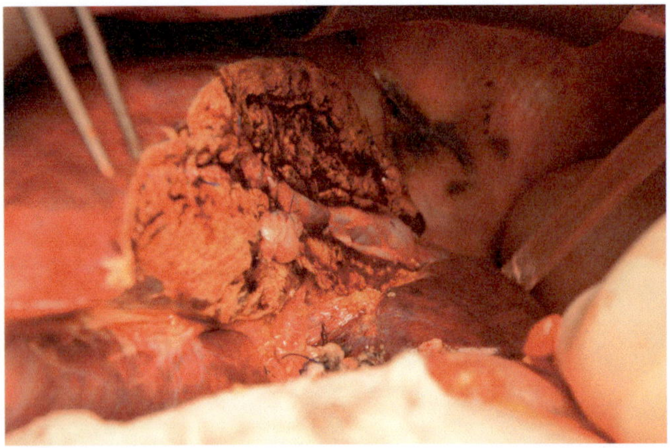

Fig. 9.21 G15678-MHV: the middle hepatic vein has been reconstructed

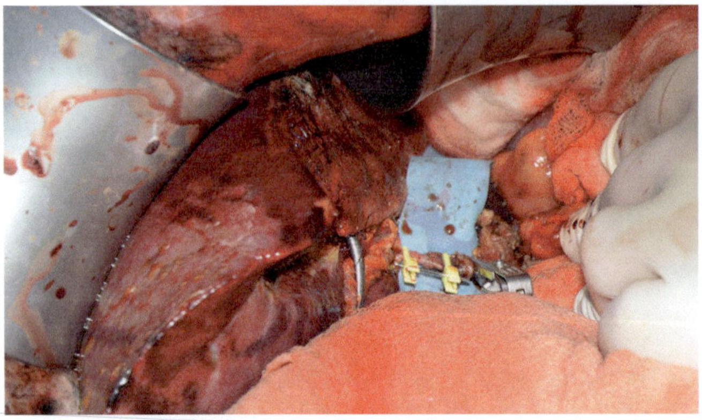

Fig. 9.22 Arterial anastomosis between the graft right hepatic artery and the native right hepatic artery

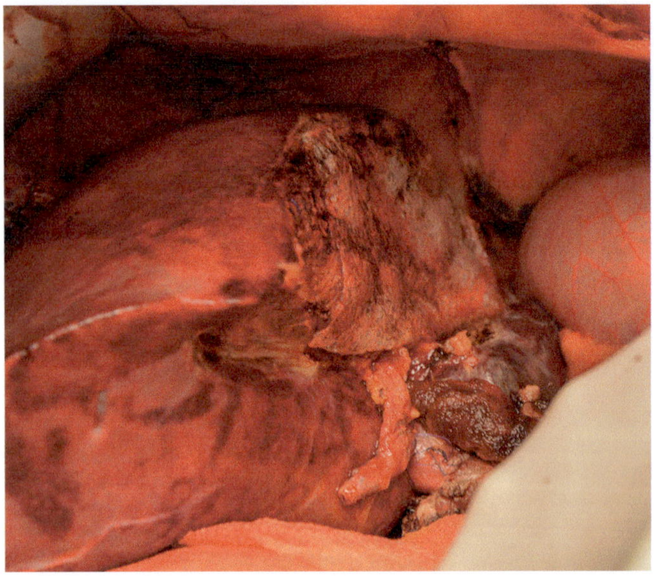

Fig. 9.23 Arterial anastomosis between the graft right hepatic artery and the native right hepatic artery after unclamping

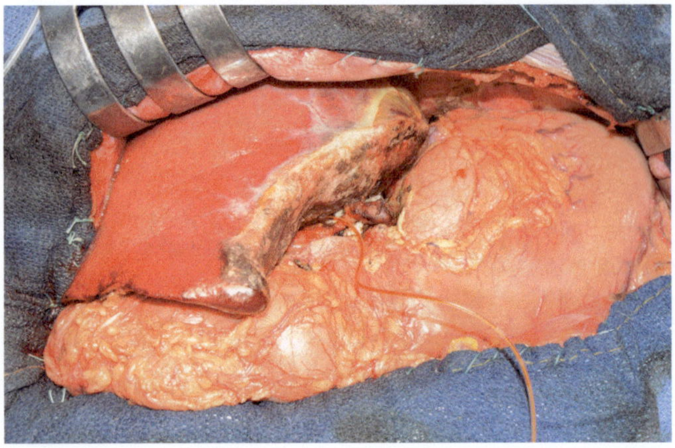

Fig. 9.24 Global view of a G15678

References

1. Azoulay D, Astarcioglu I, Bismuth H, Castaing D, Majno P, Adam R, et al. Split-liver transplantation. The Paul Brousse policy. Ann Surg. 1996;224(6):737–46; discussion 746-8. https://doi.org/10.1097/00000658-199612000-00009. PMID: 8968228.
2. Boulanger N, Muller X, Dondero F, Golse N, Goumard C, Breton A, et al. Right ex-situ split grafts for adult liver transplantation: a multicenter benchmarking analysis. Ann Surg. 2024. https://doi.org/10.1097/SLA.0000000000006401.

10 Surgical Management of Spontaneous Portosystemic Shunts

The prevalence of spontaneous portosystemic shunts is reported to be around 20–40% in end-stage liver disease patients undergoing liver transplantation [1]. These large spontaneous portosystemic shunts, when left in place at liver transplantation, have been associated with an increased risk of primary nonfunction and primary dysfunction, portal vein thrombosis, or encephalopathy possibly due to the so-called portal flow steal phenomenon and the subsequent decreased portal inflow to the graft. To prevent these complications, some have advocated ligation or division of these large spontaneous portosystemic shunts following graft revascularization (Figs. 10.1, 10.2, 10.3, 10.4, 10.5, 10.6, 10.7, 10.8, 10.9, 10.10, 10.11, 10.12, 10.13, and 10.14).

C. Lim et al., *Atlas of Liver Transplantation*, https://doi.org/10.1007/978-3-031-85264-0_10

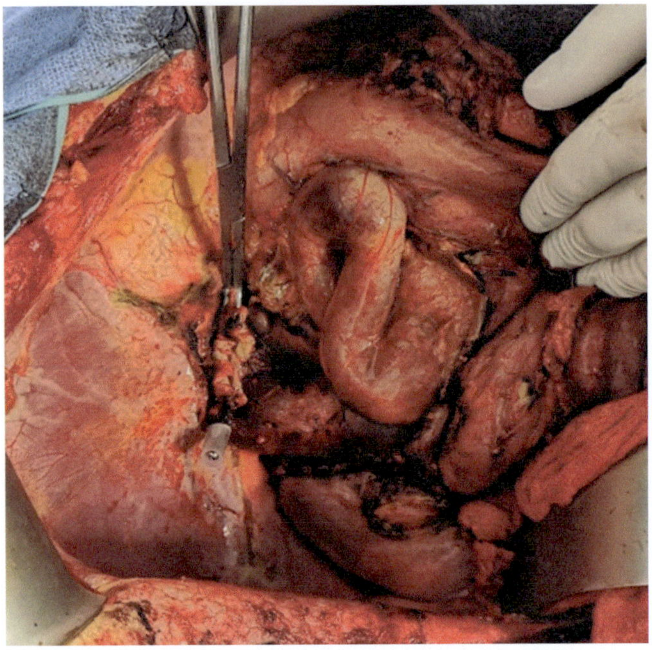

Fig. 10.1 A huge spontaneous left gastric vein

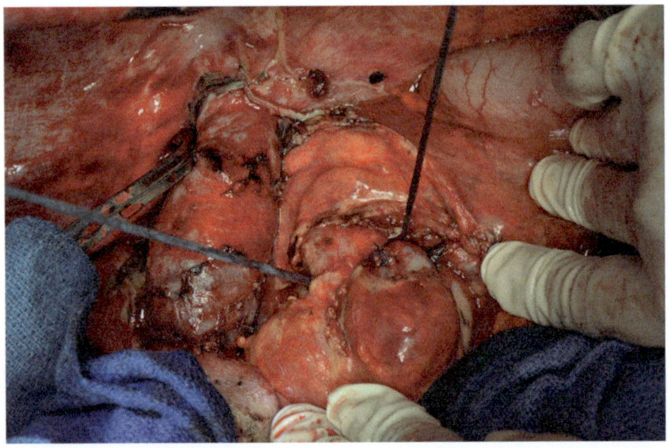

Fig. 10.2 Control of the large left gastric vein after total hepatectomy

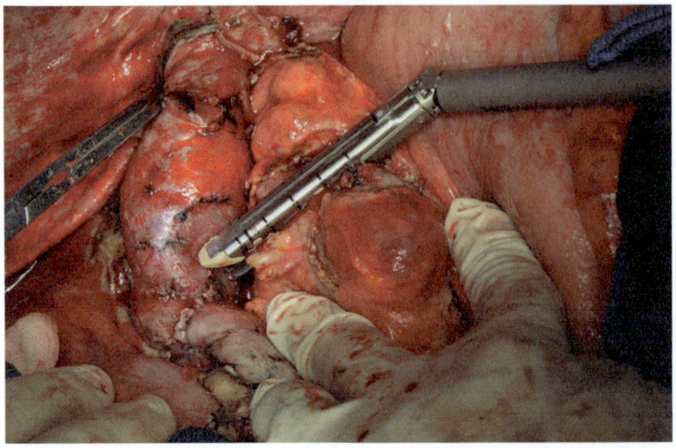

Fig. 10.3 Division of the large gastric vein using a vascular stapler

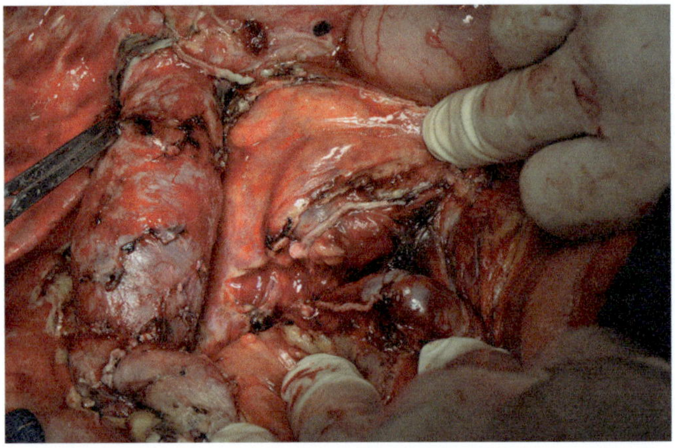

Fig. 10.4 The large left gastric vein has been divided after total hepatectomy

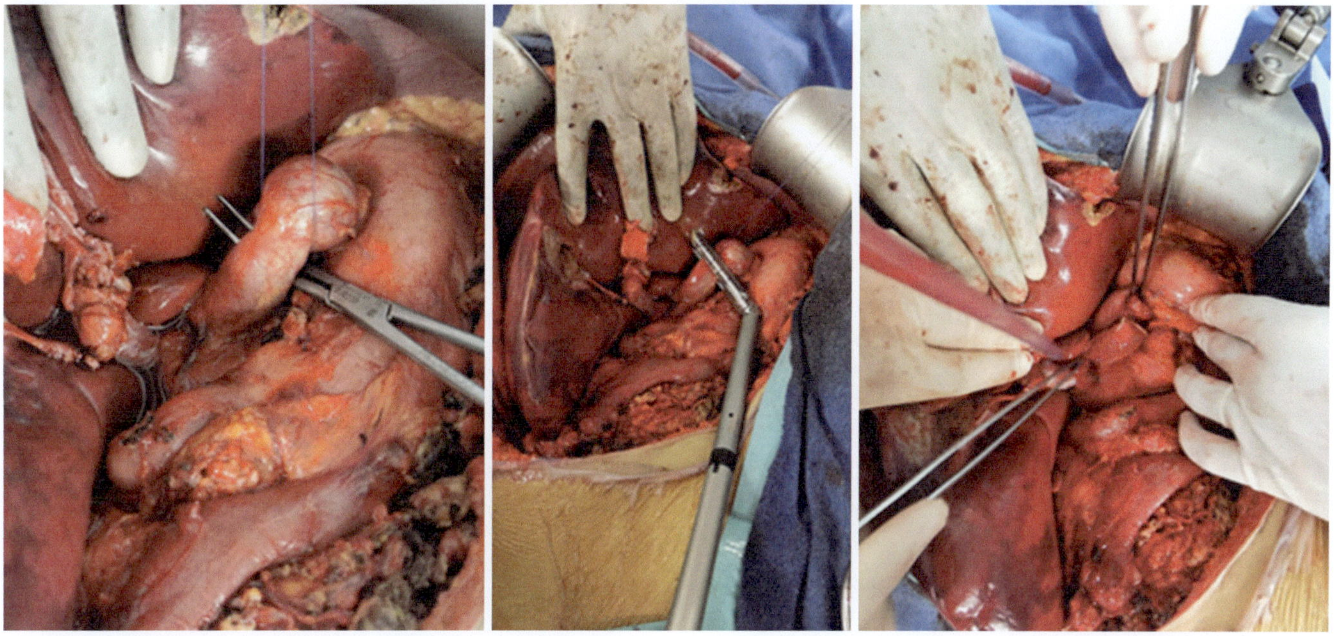

Fig. 10.5 Division of a large left gastric vein after graft revascularization

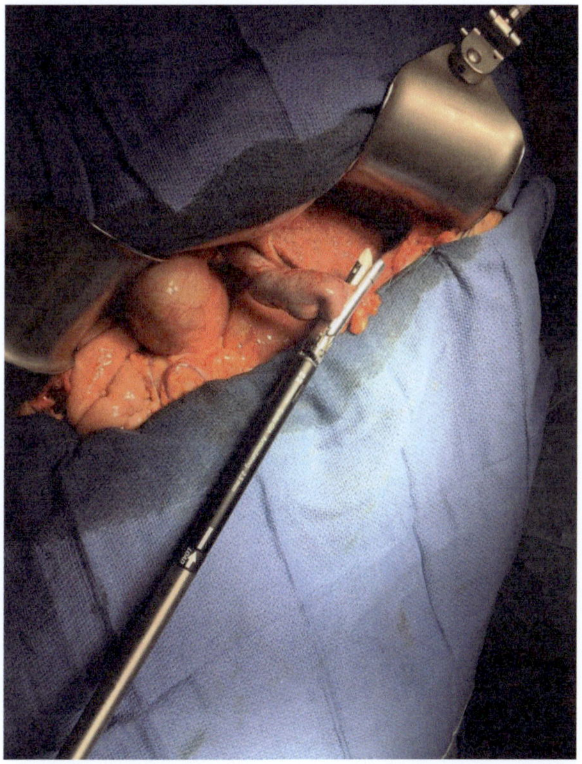

Fig. 10.6 Division of the large umbilical vein using a vascular stapler

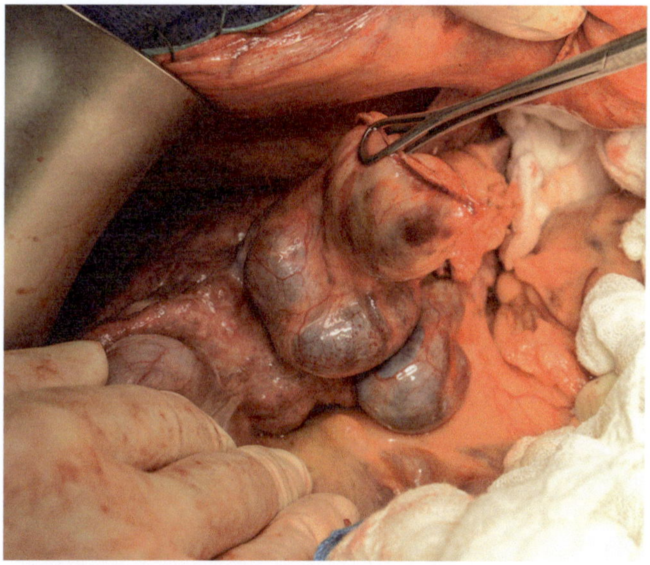

Fig. 10.7 The large umbilical vein has been divided

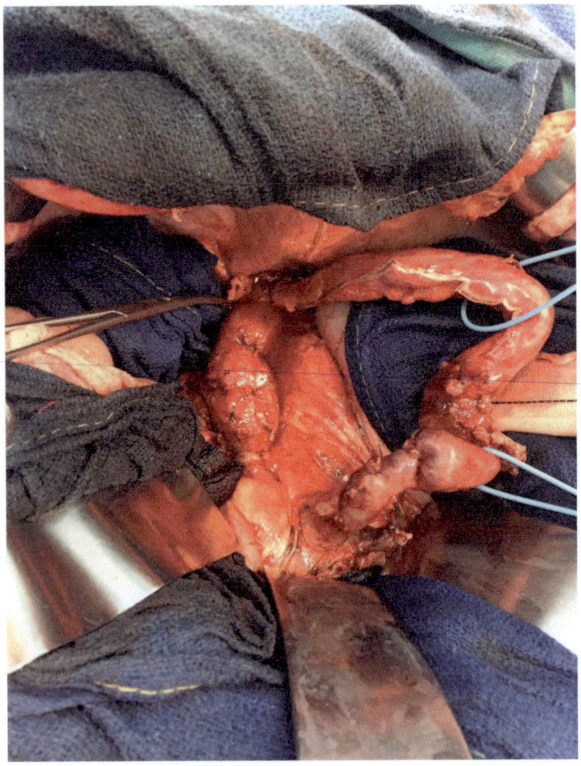

Fig. 10.8 Total hepatectomy preserving the large umbilical vein (which serves as a temporary portocaval shunt)

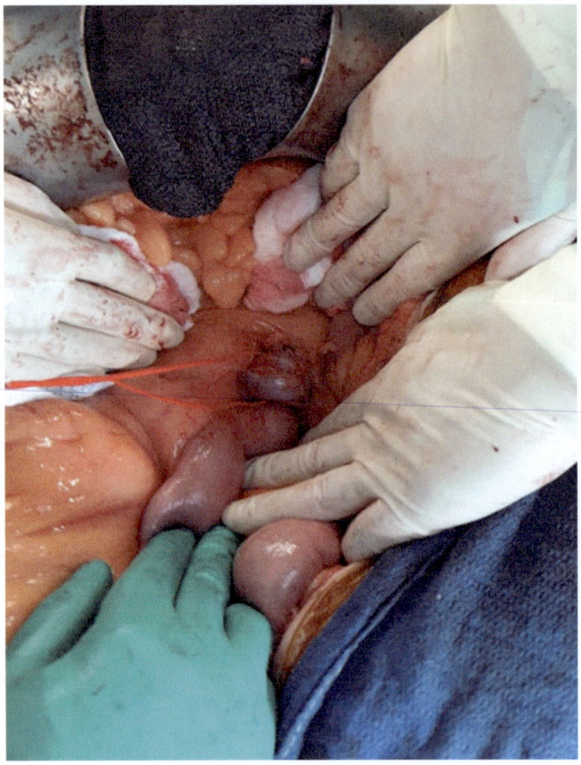

Fig. 10.10 Control of a large spontaneous mesenteric vein

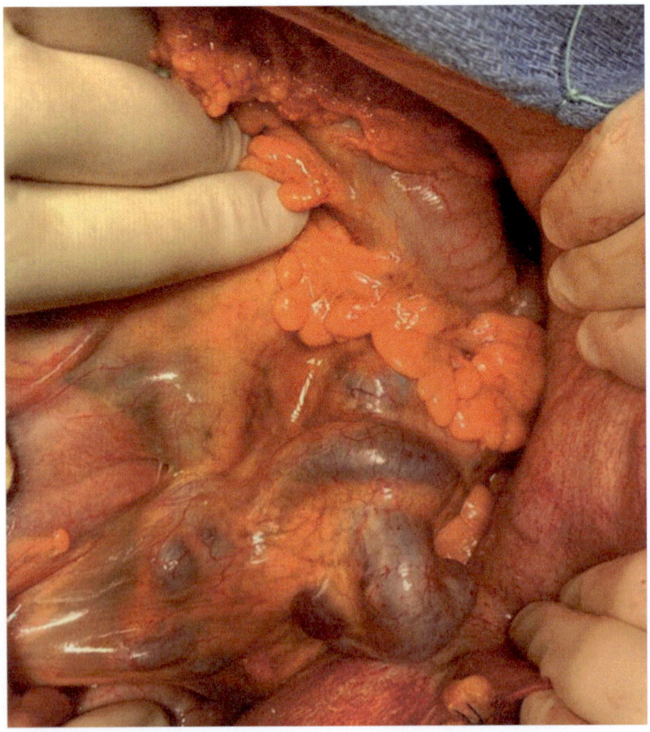

Fig. 10.9 Spontaneous and large mesenteric shunts

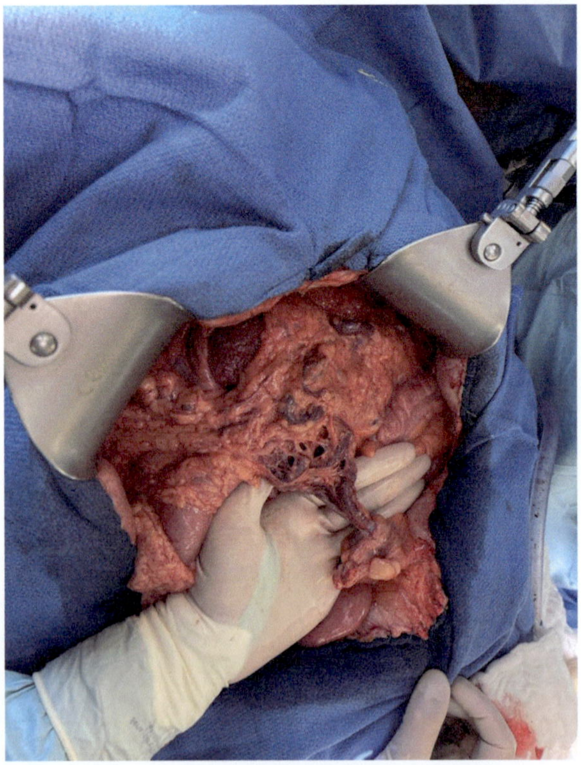

Fig. 10.11 Spontaneous and large gastroepiploic veins

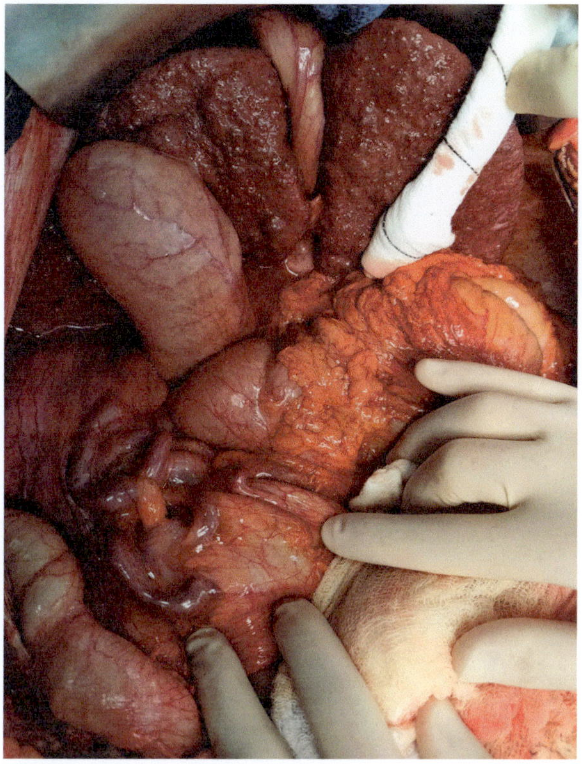

Fig. 10.12 Spontaneous portosystemic shunts between the colon and the retroperitoneal space

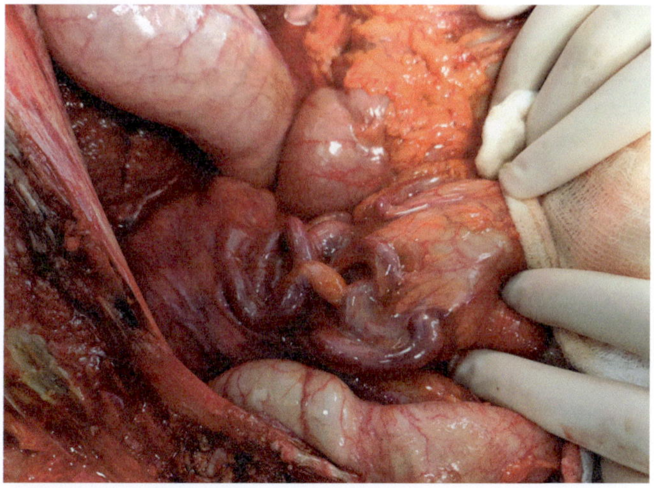

Fig. 10.13 Spontaneous portosystemic shunts between the colon and the retroperitoneal space

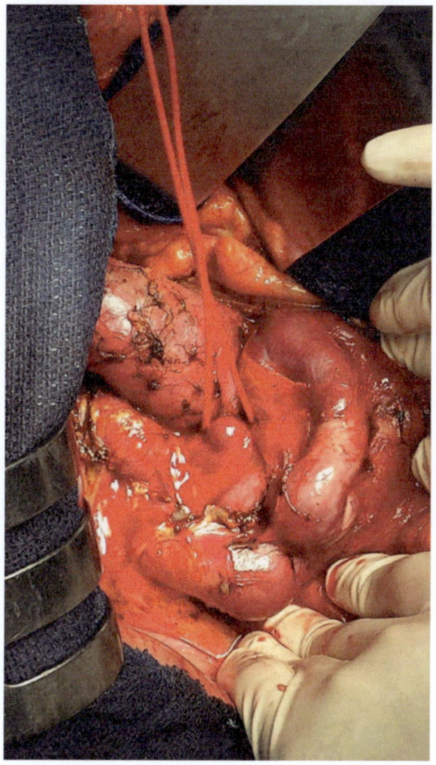

Fig. 10.14 Spontaneous mesenterico-caval shunts observed after total hepatectomy

Reference

1. Gomez Gavara C, Bhangui P, Salloum C, et al. Ligation versus no ligation of spontaneous portosystemic shunts during liver transplantation: audit of a prospective series of 66 consecutive patients. Liver Transpl. 2017;24:505–15.

11 Auxiliary Orthotopic Liver Transplantation for Fulminant Hepatitis

Auxiliary partial orthotopic liver transplantation is a procedure in which a left or right partial graft is implanted orthotopically after a native liver partial hepatectomy. In the setting of acute liver failure [1, 2], there is a possibility of recovery of the native liver and the potential for withdrawal of the liver graft (either by discontinuation of immunosuppression or surgically) (Figs. 11.1, 11.2, 11.3, 11.4, 11.5, 11.6, 11.7, 11.8, 11.9, 11.10, 11.11, 11.12, 11.13, 11.14, 11.15, 11.16, 11.17, 11.18, and 11.19).

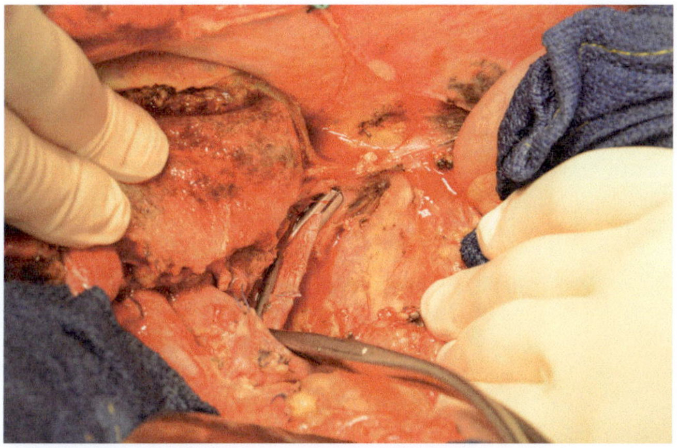

Fig. 11.1 Lateral clamping using a Satinsky forceps after left lateral sectionectomy of the native liver and removal of the caudate lobe (H123)

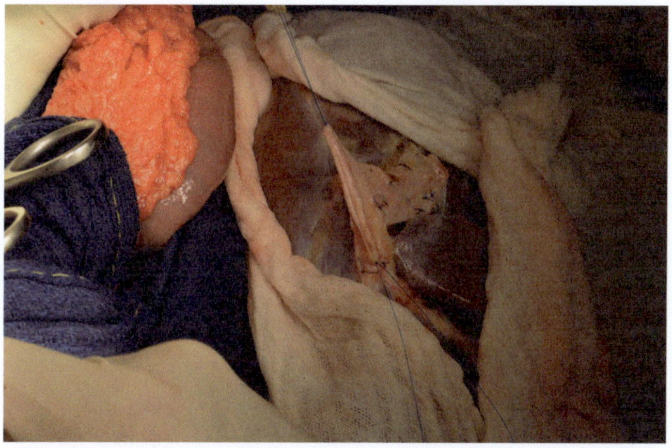

Fig. 11.2 Closure of the graft suprahepatic inferior vena cava

C. Lim et al., *Atlas of Liver Transplantation*, https://doi.org/10.1007/978-3-031-85264-0_11

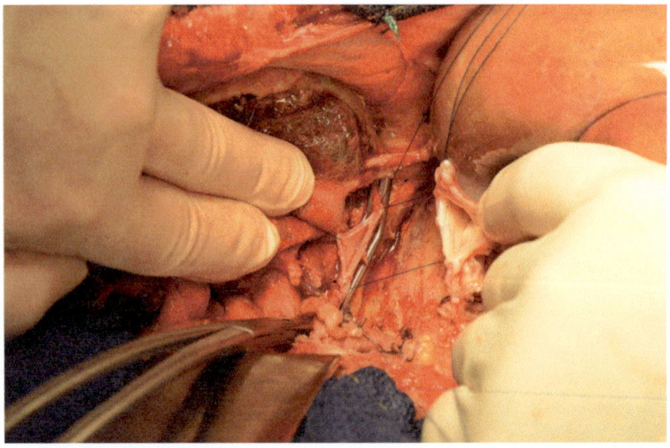

Fig. 11.3 Incision of the anterior wall of the native inferior vena cava

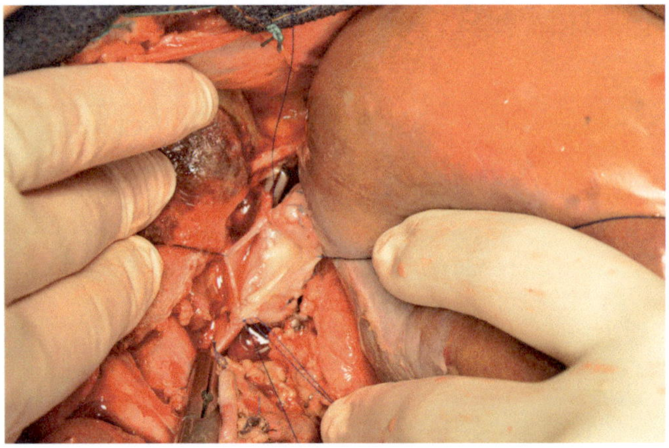

Fig. 11.4 Posterior wall of the side-to-side cavo-caval anastomosis

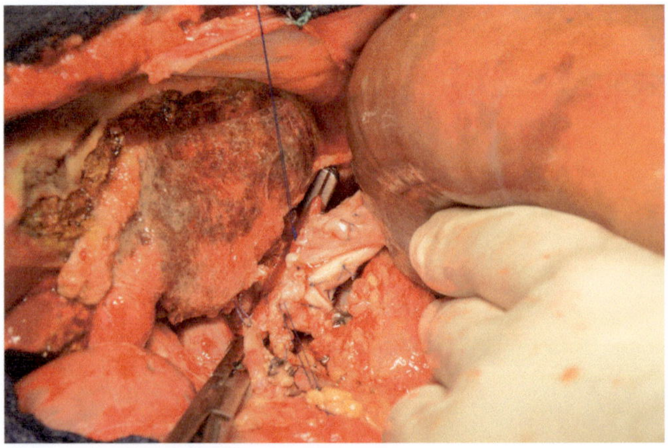

Fig. 11.5 Completion of the side-to-side cavo-caval anastomosis

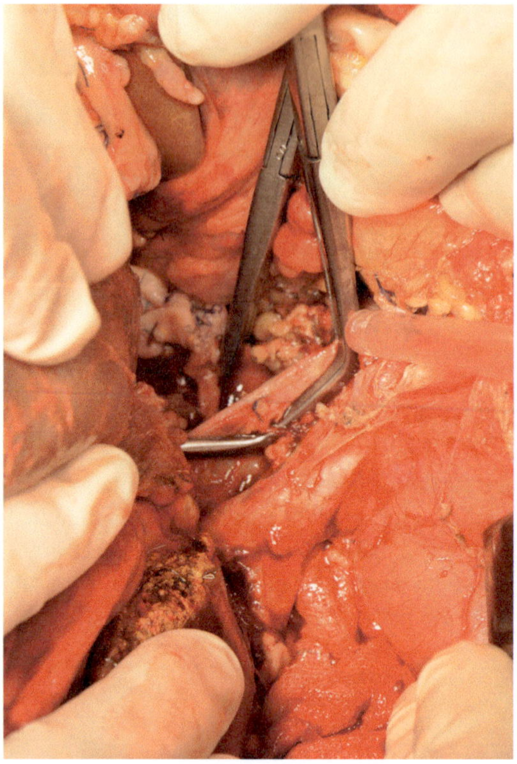

Fig. 11.6 Lateral clamping of the native portal vein

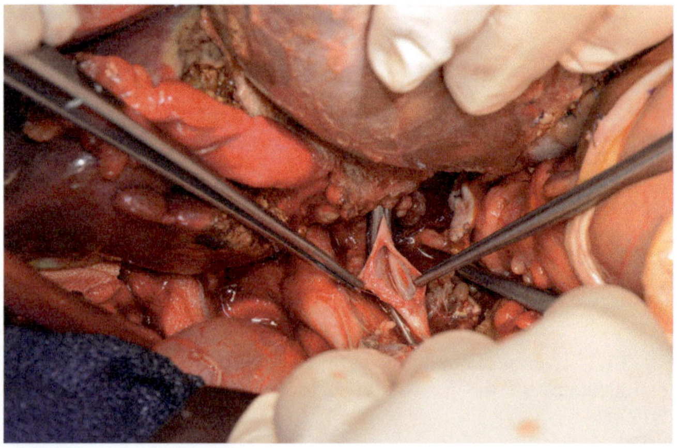

Fig. 11.7 Incision of the anterior wall of the native portal vein

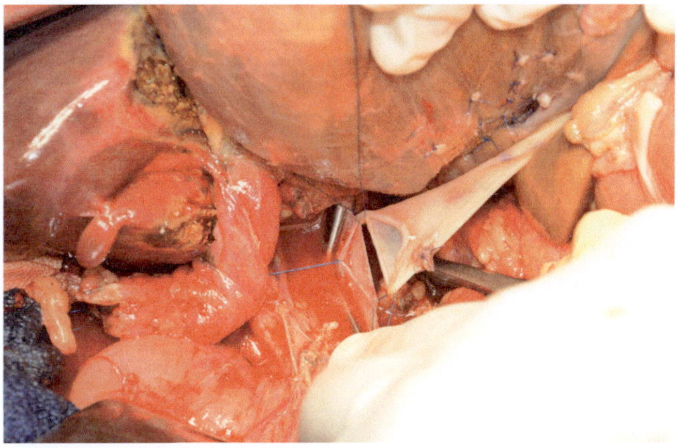

Fig. 11.8 Posterior wall of the end-to-side anastomosis between the graft portal vein and the native portal vein

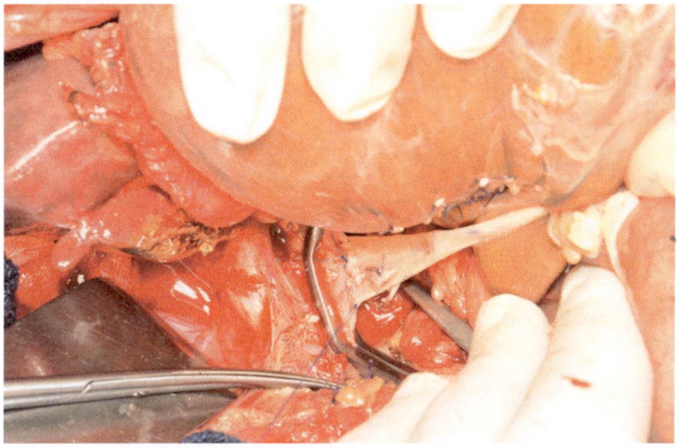

Fig. 11.9 Completion of the end-to-side anastomosis between the graft portal vein and the native portal vein

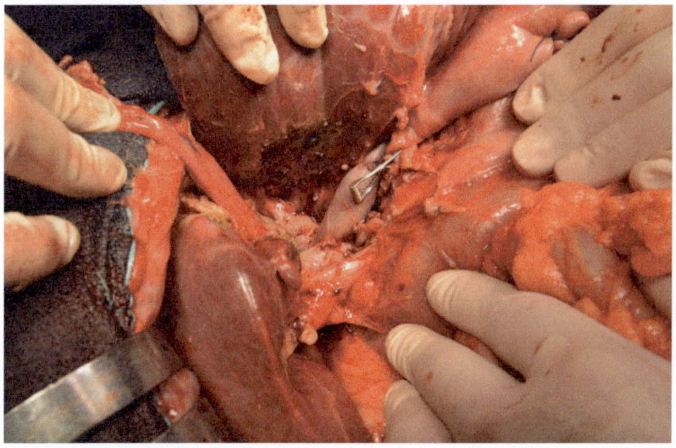

Fig. 11.10 Auxiliary whole graft revascularization

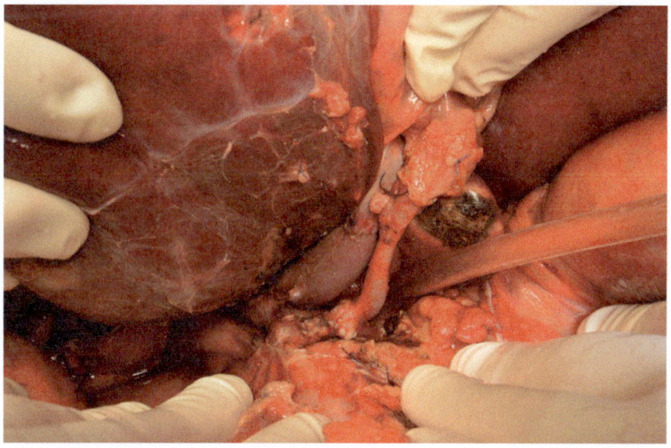

Fig. 11.11 End-to-side arterial anastomosis between the graft hepatic artery and the native splenic artery

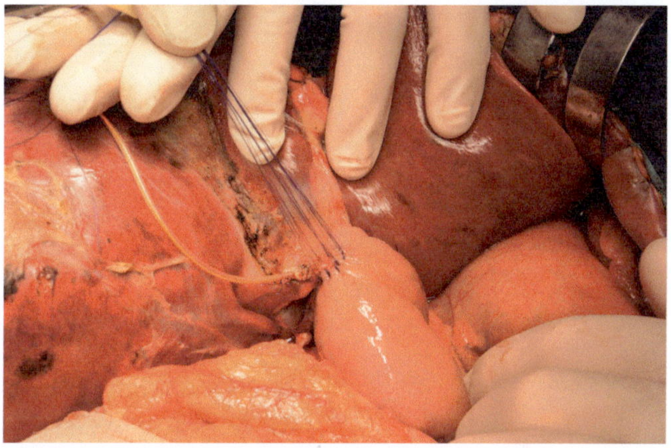

Fig. 11.12 Bilio-enteric anastomosis with an external biliary drainage

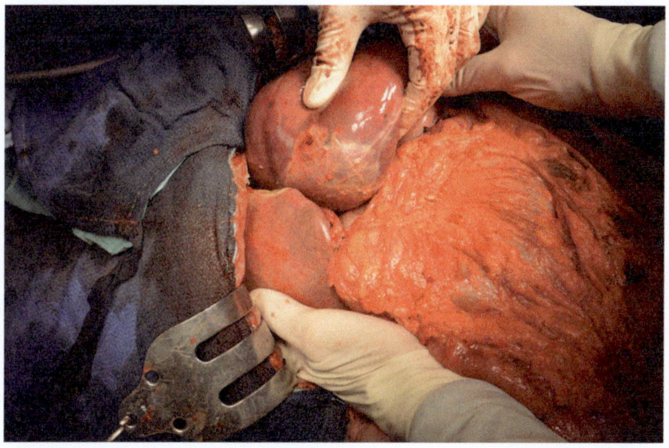

Fig. 11.13 The native liver (H45678) and the whole liver graft (G12345678)

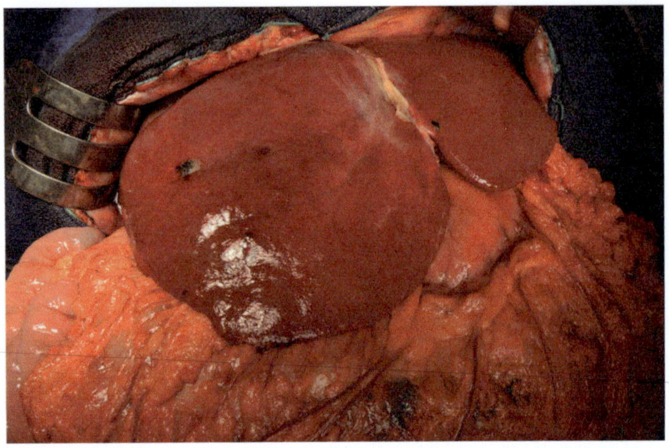

Fig. 11.14 The whole liver graft (G12345678) in the left hypochondrium

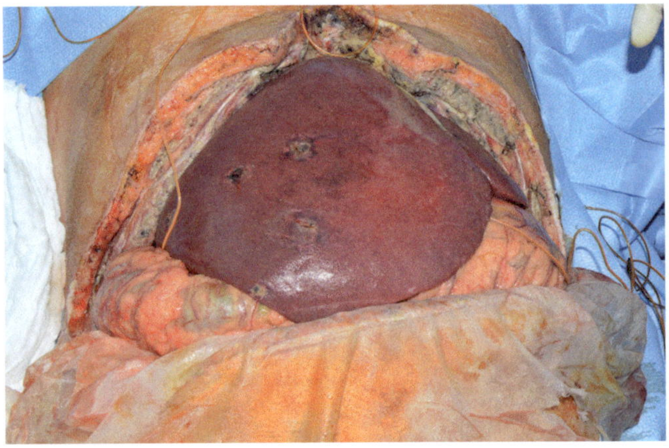

Fig. 11.15 Final aspect of the auxiliary whole liver transplantation

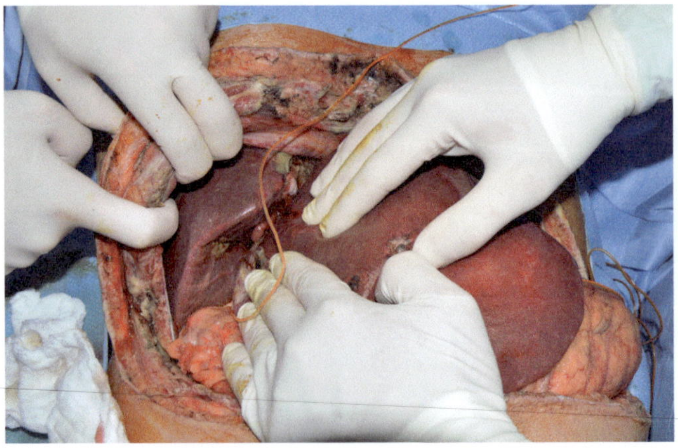

Fig. 11.16 Final aspect of the auxiliary whole liver transplantation

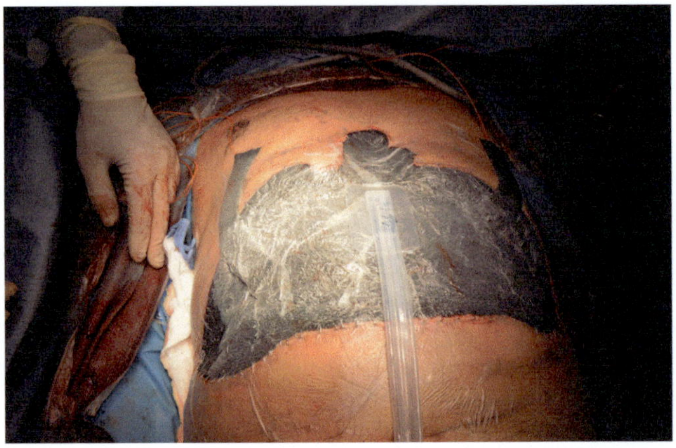

Fig. 11.17 Negative wound therapy for the management of difficult wound closure

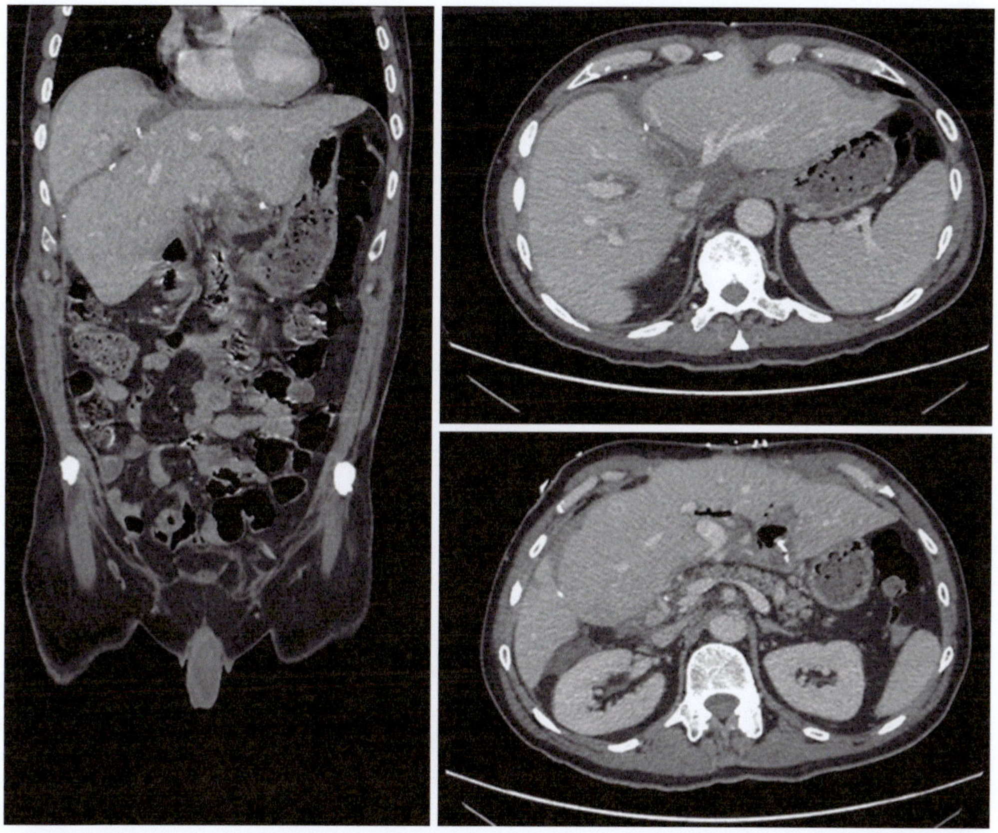

Fig. 11.18 Post-operative computed tomography (1 month)

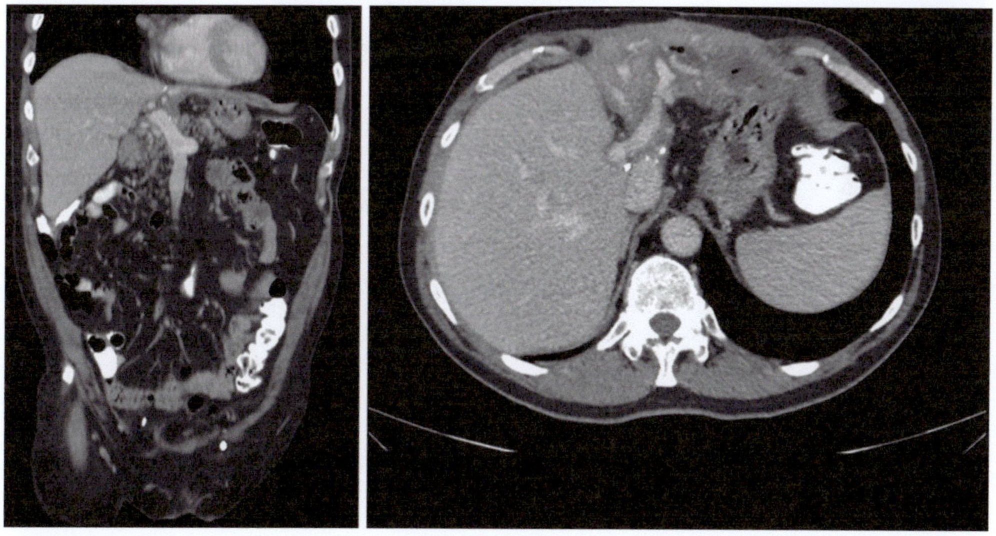

Fig. 11.19 Post-operative computed tomography after immunosuppression withdrawal (12 months)

References

1. Gubernatis G, Pichlmar R, Kemnitz J, Gratz K. Auxiliary partial orthotopic liver transplantation (APOLT) for fulminant hepatic failure: first successful case report. World J Surg. 1991;15(5):660–5; discussion 665–6.
2. Bismuth H, Azoulay D, Samuel D, Reynes M, Grimon G, Majno P, et al. Auxiliary partial orthotopic liver transplantation for fulminant hepatitis. The Paul Brousse experience. Ann Surg. 1996;224(6):712–24; discussion 724–6. https://doi.org/10.1097/00000658-199612000-00007.

12 Management of Large-for-Size Liver Graft Mismatch

Liver volume matching in liver transplantation is important. Advances have been obtained to avoid small-for-size grafts, but management of large grafts remains a major challenge in this setting. Consequences include difficult anastomosis, poor vascular alignment, difficult wound closure, graft compression, and necrosis. Negative wound therapy allows a rapid closure of abdominal wall and salvage of the graft. In addition, preservation of the native inferior vena cava using a large graft during adult whole liver transplantation is associated with potential risk of hepatic venous outflow compression/obstruction. Intraoperative placement of materials to restore adequate hepatic venous outflow can overcome this complication. Placement of inflatable materials [1] leads to gradual deflation in the postoperative period, which might obviate the need for reoperation (Figs. 12.1, 12.2, 12.3, 12.4, 12.5, and 12.6).

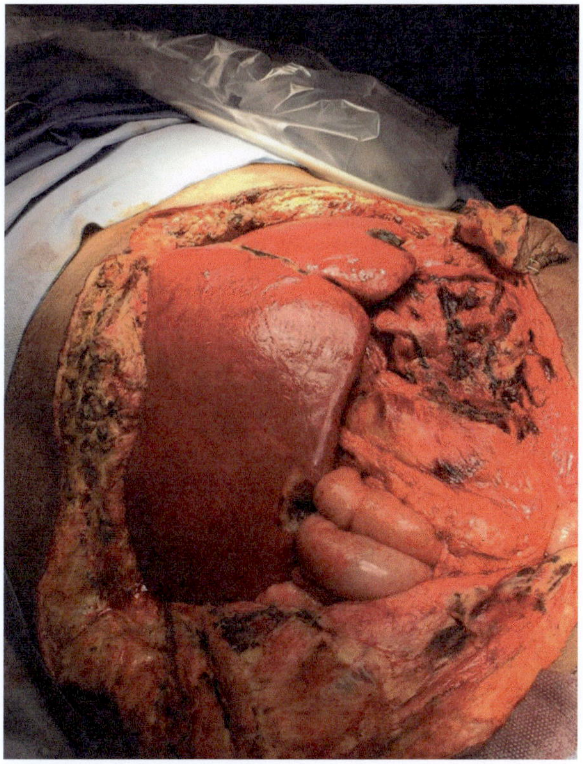

Fig. 12.1 Large-for-size liver graft

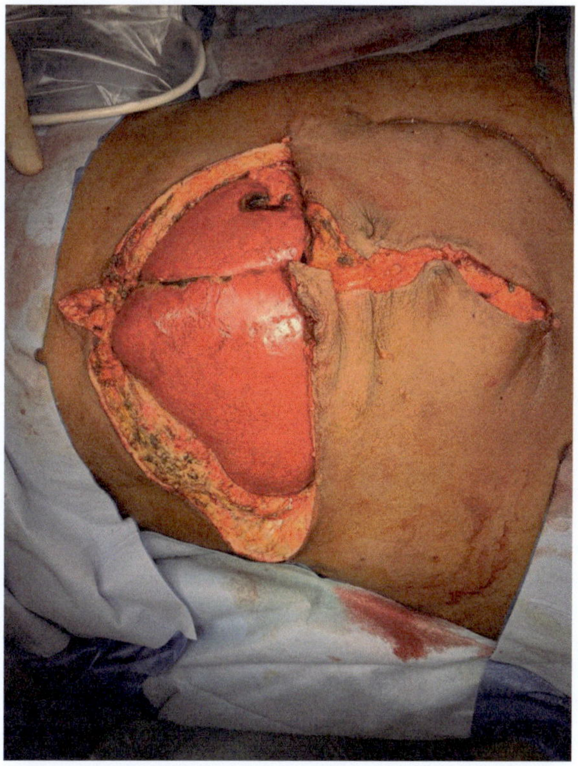

Fig. 12.2 Large-for-size liver graft after partial abdominal closure after partial abdominal closure

C. Lim et al., *Atlas of Liver Transplantation*, https://doi.org/10.1007/978-3-031-85264-0_12

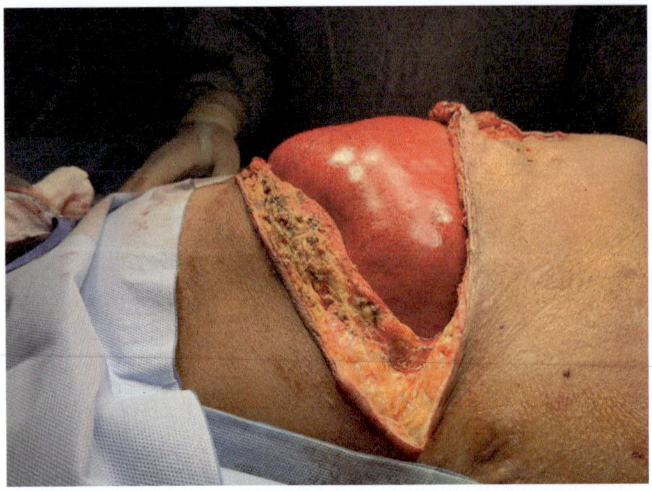

Fig. 12.3 Large-for-size liver graft after partial abdominal closure

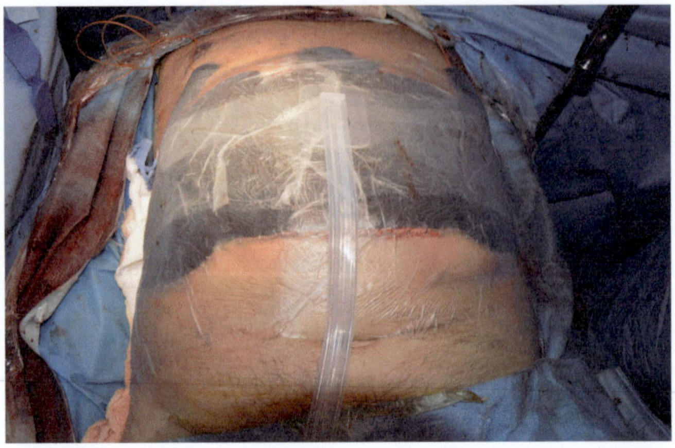

Fig. 12.5 Negative wound therapy for the management of difficult abdominal closure

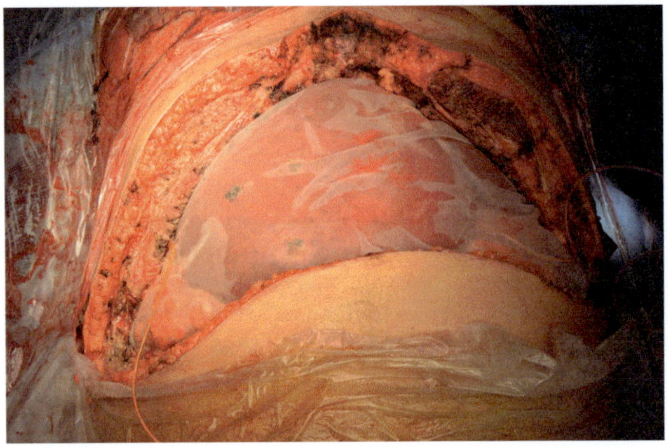

Fig. 12.4 Negative wound therapy for the management of difficult abdominal closure

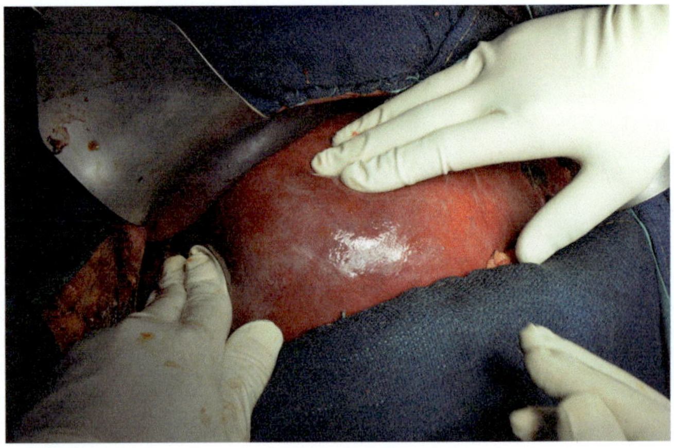

Fig. 12.6 Retro-hepatic placement of breast implants to improve hepatic vein outflow

Reference

1. Lim C, Osseis M, Tudisco A, Lahat E, Sotirov D, Salloum C, Azoulay D. Hepatic venous outflow obstruction after whole liver transplantation of large-for-size graft: versatile intra-operative management. Ann Hepatobiliary Pancreat Surg. 2018;22:321–5.

Temporary Portocaval Shunt

13

During liver transplantation, clamping of the portal vein induces splanchnic venous congestion and accumulation of noxious compounds. These adverse effects could increase ischemia/reperfusion injury and subsequently the risk of graft dysfunction, especially for grafts harvested from extended criteria donors. Temporary portocaval shunt may prevent these complications and decrease blood loss [1]. This shunt is divided before portal reconstruction (Figs. 13.1, 13.2, 13.3, 13.4, 13.5, 13.6, 13.7, 13.8, 13.9, 13.10, 13.11, and 13.12).

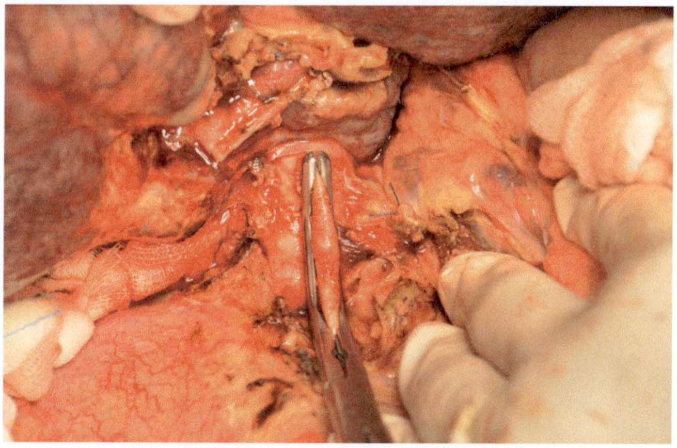

Fig. 13.1 Lateral clamping of the native infrahepatic inferior vena cava

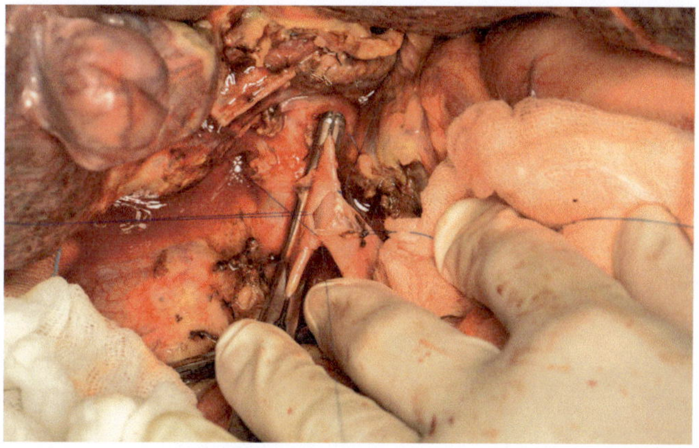

Fig. 13.2 Posterior wall of the end-to-side anastomosis between the portal vein and the inferior vena cava

C. Lim et al., *Atlas of Liver Transplantation*, https://doi.org/10.1007/978-3-031-85264-0_13

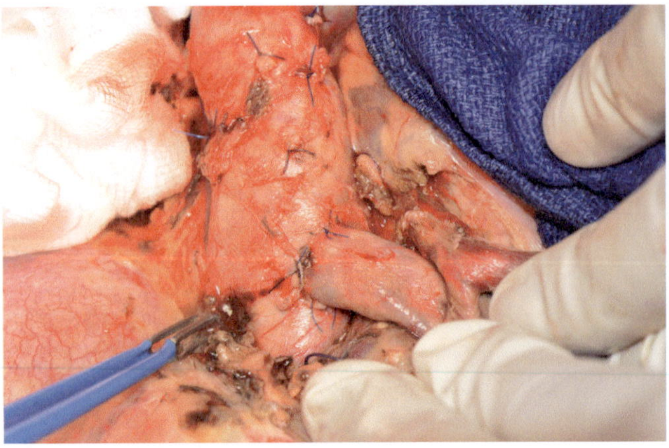

Fig. 13.3 Completion of the portocaval shunt

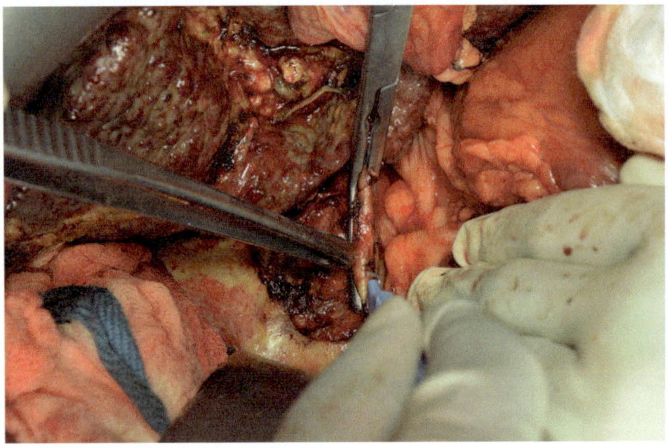

Fig. 13.4 Incision of the anterior wall of the native infrahepatic inferior vena cava

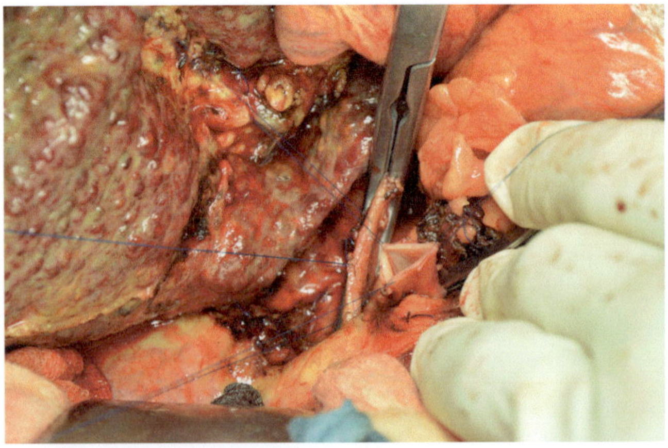

Fig. 13.5 Posterior wall of the end-to-side anastomosis between the portal vein and the inferior vena cava

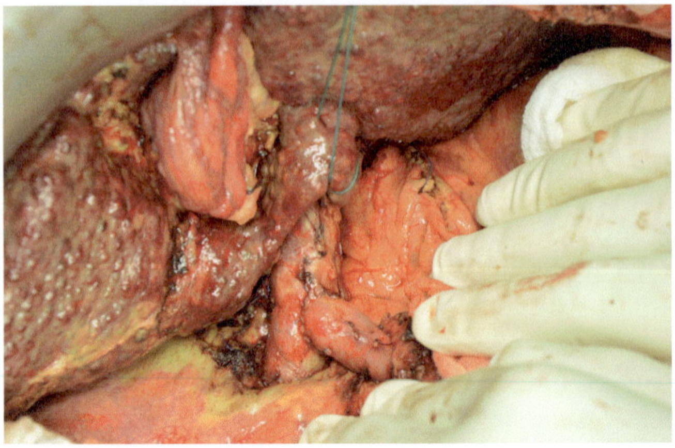

Fig. 13.6 Temporary portocaval shunt

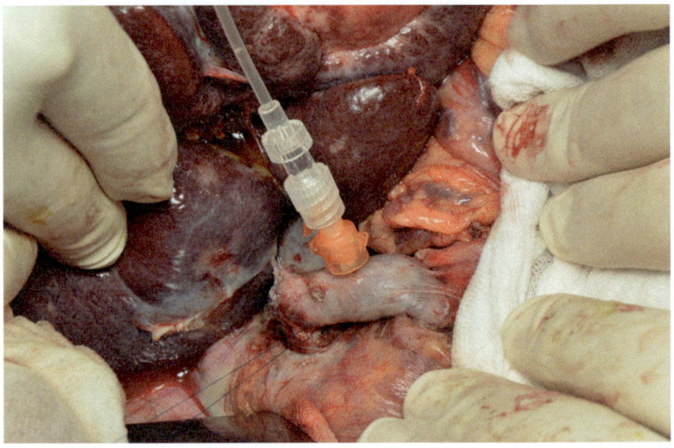

Fig. 13.7 Portal pressure measurement

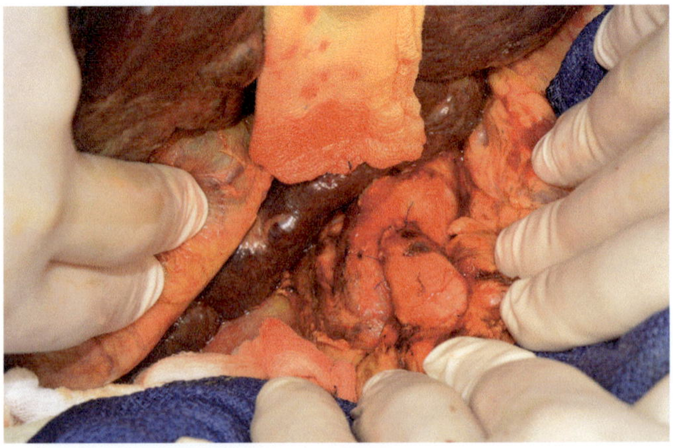

Fig. 13.8 Temporary portocaval shunt

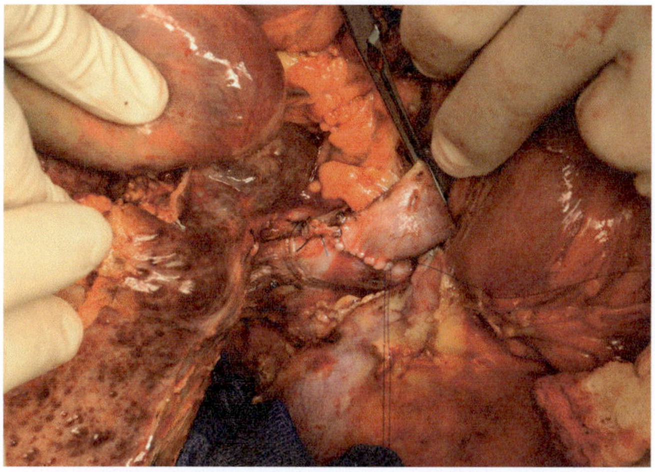

Fig. 13.9 Temporary portocaval shunt

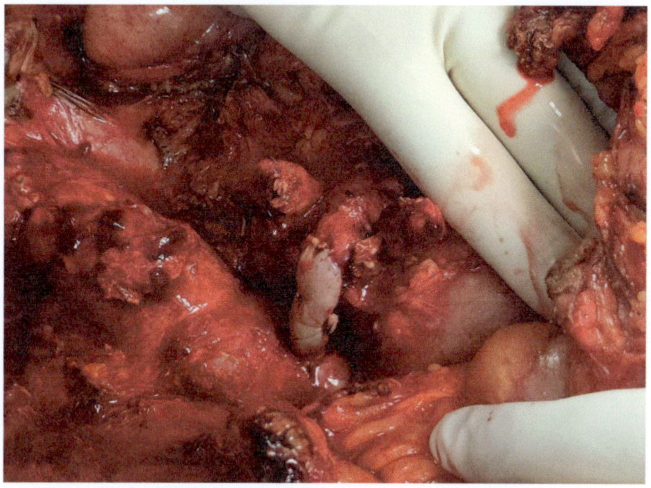

Fig. 13.11 Temporary portocaval shunt using a venous allograft because the portal vein was too short

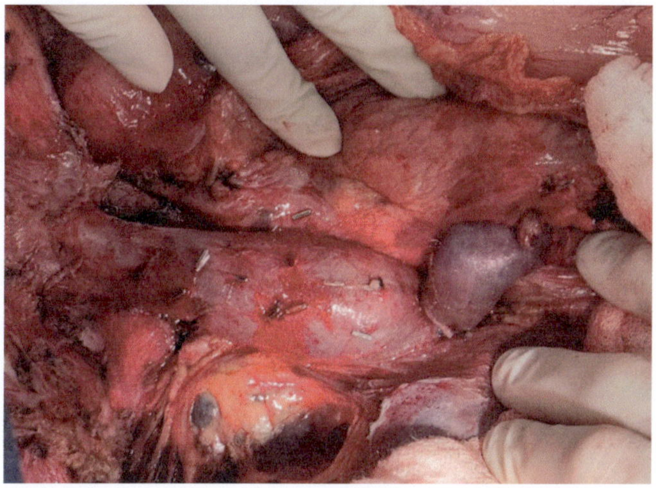

Fig. 13.10 Surgical view of a temporary portocaval shunt after total hepatectomy

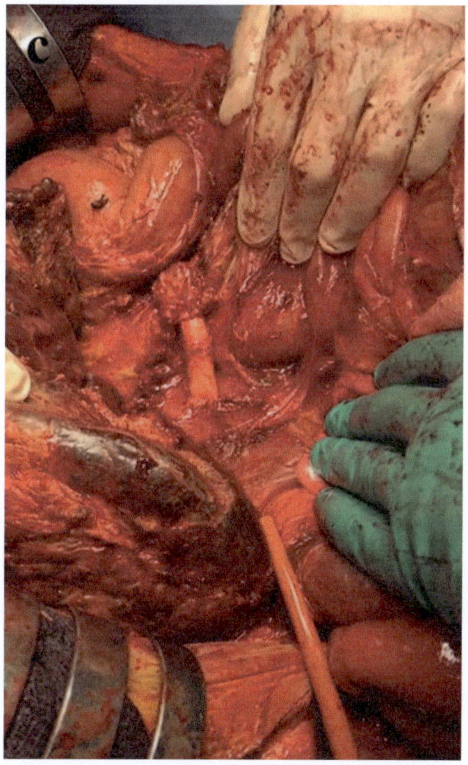

Fig. 13.12 Temporary portocaval shunt using an arterial allograft

Reference

1. Tzakis AG, Reyes J, Nour B, Marino IR, Todo S, Starzl TE. Temporary end to side portacaval shunt in orthotopic hepatic transplantation in humans. Surg Gynecol Obstet. 1993;176(2):1802.

MIX
Papier aus verantwortungsvollen Quellen
Paper from responsible sources
FSC® C105338

If you have any concerns about our products,
you can contact us on
ProductSafety@springernature.com

In case Publisher is established outside the EU,
the EU authorized representative is:
Springer Nature Customer Service Center GmbH
Europaplatz 3, 69115 Heidelberg, Germany

Printed by Libri Plureos GmbH
in Hamburg, Germany